A CAREER
IN NURSING:
Is It Right for Me?

A CAREER IN NURSING:
Is It Right for Me?

Janet R. Katz, PhD, RN
Assistant Professor
Intercollegiate College of Nursing
Washington State University
Spokane, Washington

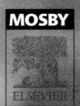

MOSBY
ELSEVIER

MOSBY
ELSEVIER

11830 Westline Industrial Drive
St. Louis, Missouri 63146

A Career in Nursing: Is it Right for Me?

ISBN-13: 978-0-323-04633-6
ISBN 10: 0-323-04633-9

Notice

Neither the Publisher nor the Author assume any responsibility for any loss or injury and/or damage to persons or property arising out of or related to any use of the material contained in this book. It is the responsibility of the treating practitioner, relying on independent expertise and knowledge of the patient, to determine the best treatment and method of application for the patient.

The Publisher

Library of Congress Control Number: 2006940678

20 06000315

Senior Editor: Yvonne Alexopoulos
Developmental Editor: Kristin Hebberd
Publishing Services Manager: Gayle May
Project Manager: Tracey Schriefer
Senior Designer: Jyotika Shroff

Working together to grow libraries in developing countries

www.elsevier.com | www.bookaid.org | www.sabre.org

ELSEVIER   BOOK AID International   Sabre Foundation

Printed in the United States of America

Last digit is the print number: 9 8 7 6 5 4 3 2 1

For Bill and Linda Katz

Preface

The purpose of this book is to help you decide whether you want to become a nurse. This is the only book you will find that discusses the profession of nursing and how to make a career decision. I decided to write this book because there was a need for it and because nursing has a history of being difficult to describe. It is important to the profession of nursing for people to understand what nurses do. It is common for people to have misconceptions about nursing that hurt the profession. Given accurate knowledge about what nurses actually do—and they do a lot—people who may not have seriously considered a career in nursing may do so. There is a worldwide shortage of nurses, and there is a need for the best and brightest to enter the nursing profession.

This book is for anyone who is considering making a career decision. If you are a student who is still in middle school or high school, this book is for you. You will also want to read it if you are in college or even if you have graduated from college and are considering or interested in learning more about a nursing career. Some people go into nursing straight from college, but many others return to college to make it a second career. The average age of a nursing student is around 32 years old.

Nursing is known for "helping people." Helping people is one way to say that nurses are advocates. Nurses take up the cause of those who need help and/or can't advocate for themselves. It just so happens that these are often children, women, people with few resources, and in the U.S., people of color, or from cultures that are different from the dominant one. Advocacy is a major part of being a nurse, and it occurs on many levels. For instance, in an emergency department or in a community health setting, a nurse may advocate for a victim of domestic violence. Advocacy is also the principle that guides this book. I am advocating for health care and—specifically—for nursing. I am also advocating for you; to try to help you make the best and most informed decision you can make.

The tone of the book is humorous because many things in nursing are not very humorous. The more serious a profession or pursuit, the more humor is needed. I use this approach as a way to make the book readable. It is my hope that by making this book readable, it can serve as a personal guide to help you understand what the nursing profession is all about and whether it is the right choice for you.

This book is organized to give you a complete picture of nursing. It begins by going over some of the common reasons people give for becoming—or not becoming—a nurse. Many of those reasons are related to myths about nursing. Next, the classes you need to take to prepare for nursing are covered. From there, the book moves through various levels of nursing school through graduation and entrance into the workplace. The book provides numerous examples of real-life nurses to help you form a picture of nursing that might be different than what you expect. The nurses who generously gave their time to talk to me and share their stories did so because they wanted others like you to understand the reality, not the myth, of nursing. Nurses contribute a vast wealth of expertise to the health care and well-being of people around the world. If after you read this book you choose this profession, you will never regret it.

Janet R. Katz

Contents

A CAREER
IN NURSING:
Is It Right for Me?

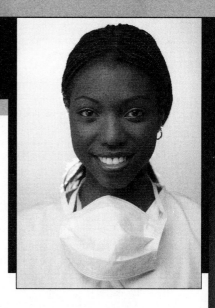

You Don't Have to Like Blood to be a Nurse

I'm a registered nurse. Often when I tell someone this, they say, "Oh, I could never be a nurse. I hate blood." Well, guess what? So do I. Nursing is about so much more than blood, and it is the "much more" that I'll be telling you about in this book. You probably have an idea of what a nurse does, but unless you have a family member or close friend who not only is a nurse but talks about being a nurse, your idea is probably incomplete. This book will help you get a realistic picture of what being a registered nurse (RN) is all about.

There are good and bad things about being a nurse and as with all decisions, you need to weigh the Pros and Cons. I suggest you keep a running list as you read this book. Make two columns. Write *Pros* at the head of one and *Cons* at the head of the other. These Pros and Cons are personal; they belong to you, so it doesn't matter what other people such as school counselors, family, or friends think. When I write about how nurses need excellent communication skills and you're thinking about how you don't really like to talk to people, include that in your Con list. If you want to be less black-and-white about it, make your list with three or four columns marked Super Pro, Pro, Con, and Super Con. In this way, you can rate the degree, or weight, of each item.

Be honest with yourself. Not everyone is going to make a great nurse, but at least give yourself the time to consider this rewarding and versatile career.

WHAT IS A NURSE?

There are as many answers to that question as there are nurses because nursing covers a lot of ground. Nurses work in so many different circumstances doing so many different things that it is hard to say that any one, two, or three things define what a nurse does. And this is exactly what makes nursing such an exciting profession. Nursing is filled with moments that are profoundly meaningful and at the same time difficult to measure or describe. How do you talk about the healing power of holding a hand? Or about an Emergency Department (ED) nurse who thinks it takes more skill to talk with a rape victim than to save the life of a trauma victim? How can nurses talk about saving lives when the doctor walks in, either in real life or on television, and gets all the credit?

Thus, it is not easy to tell someone what a nurse is, but the World Health Assembly in Geneva has done a fantastic job of answering that question. They called nurses "indispensable" contributors to worldwide national health programs and further praised nurses for their cost-effective high standards of providing quality care. Nurses were referred to as the "backbone" and the "heart" of health care who cross all geographic and political boundaries. To be internationally recognized in this way makes me proud to be a nurse.

A nursing degree can be used to work in or out of hospitals, in helicopters, on boats, and in the home. Nurses work for the U.S. Government in the military, at the National Institutes of Health, at the Centers for Disease Control and Prevention, and in Congress as representatives or senators. Nurses work internationally for relief organizations, large corporations, foreign schools, or small village clinics.

Nurses save lives, take care of people who are dying, provide pain relief, do scientific research, run hospitals, and design computer systems. With advanced degrees, nurses deliver babies, run their own clinics, provide primary care, give anesthesia to people undergoing surgery, and become lawyers in medical law. All nurses are teachers and counselors and, in one way or another, help people live healthier lives.

A few years ago, I had three jobs. The first was working in a cardiac rehabilitation center where I taught people with heart disease about exercise and lifestyle changes, the second was at a university teaching nursing students, and the third was writing for nursing publications. I loved the flexibility and as I've been writing this book, I've realized that I am doing exactly what I've always wanted to do—I'm not tied down to a nine-to-five office job. Now with a PhD I am an assistant professor. I teach half time and work on research and community service the rest of the time. I am continually learning new information, be it about health care economics, the pathophysiology of heart failure, or the psychologic impact that the diagnosis of heart disease has on a 38-year-old. I love knowing that I could quit my job and find another, although that is unlikely because I love what I do now. But what I especially love and cherish is how much I have grown as a person since becoming a nurse. I've learned more about what it means to be human than anything else, and I am grateful to the many different people who have taught me this.

I've been a nurse for 23 years and, just so you know, I haven't always been so enthusiastic about nursing. Being a nurse is hard; there have been times when I wanted nothing more than to get out of nursing. Along the way, I had to take a good, hard look at what I was doing and ask myself why I wanted to quit.

To begin with, at that time I'd only worked in a hospital, and I began to realize that I didn't like working there anymore. I was also discouraged because nursing is primarily a woman's profession. Because of this, nurses tend to be underpaid for their work, although the salary is increasing (full-time working women's earnings are 77% of men's; that's up 2% from 1998). In addition, caring for people does not have high status in our society. Compare caring, what nurses mainly do, with curing, what doctors mainly do, and you'll see which is the highest paid and carries the most prestige. "Aha," I said to myself, "you want to quit nursing because of what others think about it." It dawned on me that I wanted to quit a hard job because others didn't necessarily see its value, even though I knew it was valuable and, in fact, even essential to human life.

But, when I delved further inside myself, I knew that nursing, and the work nurses did, were incredibly unique, valuable, and, most of all, needed. This completely changed my mind. I can tell you now that nothing gets my attention like seeing there is something I can do that truly makes a difference—I don't care what anyone thinks.

I struggled with my choice to be a nurse and eventually made the decision to remain one. Doing this has strengthened my commitment to the profession, and I think it has qualified me to help you understand what nursing is and what it is not. Promoting nursing is something of a mission for me, partly because I believe in nursing's valuable service and partly because I don't want nursing care, as traditional women's work, or as just being about caring, to be thought of as second best and brushed aside. Nurses are remarkable people, and the work they do is incredibly complex, beneficial, and full of healing power. As public recognition of these qualities increases, equitable salaries and prestige will follow.

Nurses Are Not Doctor Wannabes

I can guarantee you that every nurse has heard the following at one time or another: "Why didn't you go on to be a doctor?" "You're so smart; you should be a doctor." "You're just a nurse. Are you going to become a doctor?"

The truth is that, while these assumptions may be humiliating, degrading, and hurtful, they also indicate the extent of the misunderstanding that exists about nursing. Can you imagine the reverse? "Doctor, why didn't you go on to be a nurse?" "You're so smart; you should become a nurse." "You're just a doctor. When are you going to become a nurse?" or, best of all, "Doctor, you're so good with patients. You should be a nurse!" The absurdity of these statements makes them quite laughable, but asking a nurse the same questions is not at all out of the ordinary (much less funny) and is a good indicator of how our society sees nurses.

Nurses are often viewed as being beneath doctors, not as different or equal, but as a step lower on the health profession or medical ladder. But nursing is as different from being a doctor as being a physical therapist is from being a pharmacist or as being a teacher is from being a guidance counselor—teachers and guidance counselors both work in the field of education but with different roles and licensing requirements; nurses, doctors, pharmacists, and physical therapists also work in the same field doing different kinds of work with unique licenses.

Nurses do not practice medicine; they practice nursing. They do not work in the medical field; they work in health care. Nurses have their own philosophy, theory, and concerns just as doctors and pharmacists have theirs.

The focus of nursing is on the care and health of patients, whereas the doctor's focus is on diagnosis and cure. This is a big difference. If you're interested in diseases, their causes, and how to get rid of or cure them, medicine might be for you. If you're more interested in working and caring for people to help them regain or maintain their health, nursing might be your field.

However, the two professions do overlap—often doctors care and nurses cure. You see nurses diagnosing an ear infection and writing a prescription for an antibiotic to cure that infection just as you see a doctor provide comfort and care by quietly holding the hand of a dying patient. For instance, nurse practitioners both cure and care. They work under their own license, as opposed to physician assistants who work under a doctor's license; they may write prescriptions; and they care for their own patients.

Please keep this in mind. You must analyze what each health profession does and then ask yourself: Is this what I want to do? Do not pick nursing as a career that's second best to being a doctor. Choose nursing because it lets you do what you want to do and not because of what others think or because of what you don't know— *yet.*

WHAT STUDENTS MAKING CAREER CHOICES THINK

If you read research studies about what students think of nursing as a career, you'll see that few even think about it, much less go into it. In a study of high school sophomores, less than 28% of those planning to attend college considered nursing as a career option, and of those, only 7% actually pursued it. One reason for these low numbers is that nursing is often not presented to students as a choice; if it is, it is misrepresented.

The top six reasons students give for not considering nursing as a career are:
1. Nursing school is too difficult and costly.
2. Nursing school is too difficult and not worth it later in terms of salary and status.
3. Nurses don't receive enough respect, power, or leadership opportunities.
4. Nurses work too hard and do manual labor.
5. Nurses are not appreciated.
6. Students disliked the idea of being around people who were dying.

On the other hand, the top seven reasons students gave for considering nursing were:
1. Nurses care for and help other people.
2. Nurses work with people who have illnesses.
3. There are many professional opportunities.
4. Nurses have job security.

5. Nursing is nurturing.
6. Students surveyed liked science.
7. The profession of nursing has many personal benefits.

In short, students like the idea of caring for others, using their intelligence, and learning about science; but they want more power, less hard work, and a good salary for their efforts.

We'll talk about all of these issues in this book, but for starters, nurses make a very good salary—unless you compare them with other health professionals such as doctors, some physical therapists, and pharmacists, many of whom make more than nurses. The average income for all RNs in the U.S. is $57,784. In California it is $62,000-$74,000 per year, or $30-$36 per hour (HRSA 2006).

Nurses have a great deal of responsibility—they literally hold the lives and well-being of others in their hands—thus, although the pay is excellent in terms of providing a good living, it is not as good in terms of comparable worth. It all depends on your perspective. Start thinking about salary as one of your reasons for wanting to be or not wanting to be a nurse (add it to your Pros or Cons list). Remember that the purpose of this book is to help you make a decision about nursing as a career.

WHAT DO YOU THINK OF WHEN YOU THINK OF A NURSE?

So what do you think? What is your image of a nurse? If you are thinking of nursing as a career, it is critical that you start clarifying your concept of nursing. You don't want to miss the opportunity of a lifetime by rejecting nursing on the basis of false impressions. Likewise, you don't want to waste your time going into nursing for reasons that don't match reality.

Take a moment. When you think of a nurse, what do you see? I'll bet it doesn't take you long to come up with a picture. Maybe someone in your family is a nurse. You've certainly seen nurses in the movies or on TV. Shows like *Scrubs* and *ER* portray nurses, or at least the networks' idea of nurses, as do the real-life enactment shows such as *Rescue 911*. Maybe you, a family member, or a friend have been in a hospital. Perhaps a grandparent has had a home health nurse or has recently been in a nursing home.

Close your eyes and picture "a nurse." What does your nurse look like? Is your nurse a she or a he? Does your nurse have on a white hat and white uniform? Surgical scrubs? Is your nurse holding a gigantic dripping hypodermic syringe or a bedpan? Is your nurse dressed in street clothes with a stethoscope?

Next picture what your nurse is doing. Is she or he feeding a baby or delivering one? Obeying a doctor's orders or giving orders? Standing quietly by while a doctor or priest discusses dying with a patient and family or talking while the doctors watch? Is this nurse in a hospital or in a clinic? In someone's home or flying in a helicopter? Changing sheets or prescribing medications?

I hope you're thinking, because before we can really talk about what it takes to become a nurse, you need to know something about what a nurse is. You may already have a clear idea; if so, you're one of the lucky few.

ARE YOU CONSIDERING NURSING FOR THE RIGHT REASONS?

Rebecca Sternberg, a nursing student in her last semester of school, told me:

> I didn't really know what I was getting into when I started nursing school. I thought I'd just learn how to help people. It's turned out to be so different from that. Sure, I've learned about helping people, but I've learned so much more. And it's been a lot of hard work.

Rebecca wanted to help people, and she knew that's what nurses did. She was only partly right. She had no idea how much information about diseases, drugs, math, nursing theory, communication, and assessment she would have to learn. She almost dropped out, but, with the help of her professors and, most of all, her own determination, she worked hard, graduated, and now works as an RN in geriatrics.

Karin Anderson, a high school student who grew up in a rural area north of Spokane, Washington, wanted to be a nurse ever since she had seen Pat Port, RN, save the life of her mother and her unborn brother. Realizing that her pregnant mother was about to deliver 4 weeks' early, Karin called the local paramedics. When they arrived on the scene, they immediately saw the seriousness of the situation and called for help. Pat, an experienced and skilled neonatal nurse who worked on the mother-baby team of a helicopter ambulance service, flew out with the pilot and a respiratory therapist to Karin's home in the country. Pat stabilized her patient and successfully transported the mother into the hospital for a safe delivery.

Karin was so impressed by Pat—by her confidence, her skill, and her gentle reassuring manner—that she decided then and there that this was something she wanted to do. Karin has a long way to go to reach the level of nursing that Pat practiced, but it is not out of her reach. Like Karin, many students decide on nursing after an encounter with a real nurse in a real-life situation. They see the authority and power these nurses have, and they see nursing as something to aspire to.

Joe Adams has been a nurse for 25 years. He went into nursing after being a medic in the Vietnam War. He told me that becoming a nurse was a decision he made because of his Vietnam experiences. He wanted a career in the medical field, but not as a doctor, because he wanted to spend more time with his patients: talking, comforting, and teaching them, as well as helping them make connections when needed through community resources. He decided to work in emergency care as a nurse.

I asked him what he would tell someone who was thinking about going into nursing today. He said, "I'd tell them to think very carefully about it first."

I asked him why, and he explained,

Nursing isn't like it used to be. It's not as easy as it used to be. You have to be motivated and know what you want to do and set goals.

Then I asked him, "How can a student possibly know what she or he wants to do?" He advised, "Tell her or him to volunteer or spend a day in an area she or he is interested in—say, the ED or a health clinic."

I've heard this advice over and over from other nurses. They emphatically suggest that anyone considering nursing should observe what nurses do and talk to them. Ask nurses questions such as the following:

- How do you organize and prioritize your work each day?
- How do you know when a patient needs help?

The thinking process behind the answers to these questions is a big part of nursing, and by asking them you'll start to find out what goes on in a nurse's head and thus what the work is really about.

Spend time going to the places you are interested in. The nurses who work there will very likely welcome you. Remember to call ahead and explain that you want to see what they do in their job because you are interested in becoming a nurse.

Tell them that you want more firsthand experience so that you can be sure before you commit to the nursing profession.

Another option is to volunteer. Many hospitals, clinics, and nursing homes have volunteer positions. Volunteering gives you an excellent firsthand look at what nurses do, as well as an opportunity to meet and talk with them.

ARE YOU AVOIDING NURSING FOR THE WRONG REASONS?

A friend of mine has a daughter who is graduating as valedictorian from high school this year. She told me that her daughter had talked about going into nursing because she wanted to work in health care and because she was interested in science and liked working with people. Even though these were perfectly good reasons for going into nursing, she decided against it because it lacked prestige. Instead she decided to become a medical technician and work in a hospital laboratory.

This is an example of deciding not to go into nursing for the wrong reasons. Although nursing may be perceived as lacking prestige, studies show that people who have been hospitalized think nurses are the most important people there. National polls consistently show that people rate nurses as the most trustworthy professionals, above doctors and lawyers. To the people who have been cared for by a nurse, the nurse is a problem solver, a comfort giver, a skilled troubleshooter, and a real lifesaver. Don't forget that nursing's image is changing. Nurses and their professional associations are campaigning hard to show people what nurses really do. The American Nurses Association and many others have full-time media personnel especially for this purpose.

Health care is changing as well. New nursing opportunities such as nurse practitioner, midwife, and researcher are growing roles. The prestige and authority of nursing is changing and growing just as fast. This is a golden time for nursing, and, although we are having bumpy times along with the rest of health care, we are at a point of great positive change and great positive energy. This will go a long way toward improving the image of nursing that makes it seem less of an attractive career than it really is.

DO YOU KNOW WHAT YOU WANT TO BE WHEN YOU GROW UP?

It's not uncommon to never want to grow up, but that doesn't mean you don't have to decide what you are going to do for a living. It does mean that you may change careers as you go along, which is exactly what more and more people are doing these days; many people come to nursing from other careers.

However, if you are younger, you may be deciding for the first time what you want to do. In some ways it's like going fly-fishing—casting your line here and there, looking for a good spot, hoping you find one of those deep pools full of opportunity.

On the other hand, you may be able to say, "I've always known I wanted to be a nurse." If this is the case, you can use this book's advice to make sure you do so for the right reasons and to make critical decisions about your education.

If you don't know for sure, this book will go a long way toward helping you make a decision. As a nurse, I'm qualified to tell you that asking the question, "What do I want to be when I grow up?" is healthy. Asking it throughout your life puts you on a lifelong learning curve that will keep your mind and soul in excellent shape. And, as you know, a healthy mind promotes a healthier body.

Your assignment, then, is to think about your concepts of nursing, the images of nurses you see portrayed on TV and in books. Compare them with reality. Then think about whether you want to be a nurse. Start out with the following exercise. Make a list, or draw a picture, of your typical nurse. Consider the gender, age, personality, and type of work your nurse is doing. Don't forget to include what you think and feel about all of this. For example, your nurse might be carefully assisting an elderly person with his or her insulin injections. Do you think of this in a positive way?

ANGELS OF MERCY AND OTHER MYTHICAL CREATURES

Nursing is not short of one thing: stereotypes. Examples include Florence Nightingale as an angel of mercy; the sexy war nurse, just as Hemingway may have pictured her, on the cover of pulp paperbacks; or a vindictive sneering Nurse Ratched harassing Jack Nicholson in the famous 1975 movie, One Flew Over the Cuckoo's Nest.

One classic stereotype was conjured up in 1843 by Charles Dickens in the novel Martin Chuzzlewit. In it we are introduced to Sarah Gamp, midwife, home nurse, and "layer-out of the dead." She was mainly a comic figure; but she was also uneducated, unprincipled, and a drunk. The image of Sarah Gamp the nurse remains alive today and is considered by nursing historians a frighteningly accurate portrayal of the mid–19th century nurse. Others give the Sarah Gamps of the 19th century more credit by arguing that these nurses practiced their profession independently and were far more clinically proficient than physicians of the day. Whether the portrayal of Sarah Gamp is historically accurate or not, it certainly underscores how fictional characters can affect our thinking.

Stories about women have frequently centered on male characters, romances, and marriages, while neglecting personal achievements and rewards. Nurses are no exception and indeed have provided ample fodder for the pulp fiction mill. Nurses are portrayed in gender and sexual conflicts, as mothers, sisters, sexual temptresses, or, in the reverse, as lonely, cold spinsters who work solely to fill the void of an unhappy life. Rarely are they portrayed as proficient, educated, caring professionals.

The depiction of nurses in fiction shows how our culture regards them. Many stories portray nurses first as vulnerable women and second as skilled workers. One of my personal favorites is a paperback titled Affairs of a Ward Nurse (Born to be Bad [1964] Belmont) by Mitchell Coleman with the tagline "The flaming history of a nurse who was a woman first!" This, of course, implies that nurses cannot do both—unlike the male doctors they fall in love with, who seem quite capable of being husbands, lovers, and saviors of humanity, all at the same time.

Another book that makes me laugh (and let me add that it has taken me a long time to appreciate the cultural significance of these books with humor, because they used to completely offend me) is called Wilderness Nurse by Marguerite Mooers Marshall (Philadelphia, 1949, Macrae-Smith-Co.). The tagline on the cover is, "A master surgeon healed both her body and her heart." That kind of thinking leads down the path of seeing nurses as virtuous and pure, who must decide between work and a life of immorality; they must not give in to desire and thereby forsake humanity. Don't forget that it is usually a doctor who is seen as the target of the young nurse's passions, but they are not seen as equally culpable or immoral.

Not all the images we see are misleading. A picture of a nurse in Vietnam, Afghanistan, or Iraq working long hours to save lives; the image of a nurse providing care and comfort in the home of a dying patient and family; or a nurse caring for a premature baby not much bigger than a fist are heroic images, very different from the ones in fiction. They show nurses doing their work for the sake of that work, not to find a husband, be a martyr, or play a bossy matron.

Before I became a nurse or even thought of becoming one, I didn't know about the heroic images; I knew only the negative stereotypes. Nursing didn't appeal to me at all, nor did it seem exciting or challenging. I had no idea what it took to be a nurse. My idea of nurses was that they wore white, followed someone else's orders, and worked with sick people in hospitals. I didn't like hospitals, I didn't like being around sick people, and I didn't want to take orders.

When I was 23, I was working as a counselor with a woman named Dale at a family planning clinic in Massachusetts. She was quitting her job as the manager of volunteers to go to nursing school, and I was shocked. Why would Dale, so smart, so down-to-earth, and independent, want to be a nurse? I never asked her that question, but I did see her again about a year later. She said she loved nursing school and was excited about being there. She looked the same, dressed the same, and talked the same. "Hmmm," I thought to myself, "maybe there is something to nursing that I don't know about."

Later that year I began working as a clinic assistant in a neighborhood health center run by nurse practitioners. These nurses were amazing; they acted so differently from my previous concepts. They completed health examinations, diagnosed problems, and prescribed treatments. They talked to the clients and answered all their questions about their illnesses and about taking care of their bodies with confidence and kindness. I never asked them any questions about being a nurse, mainly because I was shy and easily intimidated and because I thought they knew so much and I so little. But I found it all very interesting; and I began to form a new, more realistic image of nursing.

It was quite a few years later before I actually went to nursing school, but the seeds were planted back in the health center. So, you see, stereotypes can be changed by observing real nurses. One study of nursing students found that the biggest influence on their decision to go into nursing was having a family member who was a nurse. So start looking. Whom do you know, whom can you ask, or, in this case, what can you read? I'm a real nurse, and I can tell you what real nurses do.

REAL NURSES ARE REAL PEOPLE

Information such as where nurses work, what they do, who they are, and how much money they make can enhance your understanding of the nursing profession and, in turn, help you make a career decision. In this section I have included statistics on nursing demographics from the American Nurses Association, the National Bureau of Labor, the U.S. Department of Health and Human Services (HRSA), and the American Association of Colleges of Nursing.

Nursing is the largest health profession in the United States. In 2004, the most recent data, there were 2.9 million nurses in the United States. This is up from about 2.7 million in 2000. The number of nurses increased by close to 8%. This is a greater increase than between 1996 and 2000. But it is less than the increase between 1992 and 1996. The rate of growth in nursing is not enough to meet the demand.

Of these 2.9 million nurses, 83.2% are employed and working as nurses. More nurses than ever (58.3%) are working full-time; 24.8% work part-time. Over half of all nurses work in hospitals. About 56% of all nurses work in hospitals today, but that may continue to drop as more health care services are being offered in outpatient clinics, homes, community centers, and nursing homes. In the past, the first job of most newly graduated RNs was in a hospital. Now more new graduates are going to work in community settings such as nursing homes. About 15% of nurses work in public health and community health nursing, 11.5% in ambulatory care (outpatient and clinics), 6.4% in long-term care such as nursing homes, and 2.6% in nursing education. There is a shortage of nurses in all areas of practice.

The average salary for nurses in all settings is $57,784, a 12% increase since 2000. Nurses with advanced practice, or graduate, degrees can earn $80,000 to over $100,000 a year. Approximately 8.3% of all RNs work as advanced practice nurses. These include nurse practitioners, nurse midwives, clinical nurse specialists, and nurse anesthetists. Of these, 82.3% are either nurse practitioners or clinical nurse specialists. The latter title is expected to be changing to a clinical nurse leader title.

The average age of a nurse is about 47 years old. Only 8.1% of nurses are under the age of 30. The average age of a new nurse is 30 years old (HRSA 2006). Many enter nursing as a second career; close to 37% of RNs previously worked in other health care positions. Many of these RNs had other college degrees before entering nursing (National League for Nursing [NLN], 2006, Nursing Data Review).

Over 94% of nurses are women. In 2004, only 5.7% of nurses were men, but this number is growing. Nursing schools report that as many as 12% to 13% of their students are men (NLN, 2006).

Non-Caucasian RNs make up only 10.6% of all nurses: 4.6% are African-American (non-Hispanic), 3.3% are Asian/Pacific Islander, 1.8% are Hispanic, and 0.4% are Alaska Native or American Indian. As recruitment efforts increase, there will be more diversity among nurses (HRSA, 2006).

Table 1-1 shows why we need to recruit more nurses of color and nurses from different cultures. Nurses need to be culturally competent, and patients need to be able to see nurses who are like them. You can see that, even though nursing is more diverse than other health professions, it has a long way to go to reflect the U.S. general population.

Foreign-born nurses are increasing in the U. S. nursing workforce. Nurses seeking better opportunity than their home countries may offer to come to the U.S. There has been concern among nursing organizations that the U.S. is taking nurses away from their own needy countries. But, the solution is not to limit these nurses opportunities,

TABLE **1-1**	Ethnicity of Nurses Compared With the Ethnicity of U.S. Population	
Ethnicity	**U.S. Nurses (%)**	**U.S. Population (%)**
Caucasian, non-Hispanic	88.4	67.9
African-American, non-Hispanic	4.6	12.2
Hispanic	1.8	13.7
Native American/Alaska Native non-Hispanic	0.4	0.7
Asian/Pacific Islander, non-Hispanic	3.3	4.1
Two or more races, non-Hispanic	1.5	1.3

Data from Health Resources and Services Administration (HRSA 2006): *Preliminary findings: 2004 national sample survey of registered nurses*, Washington, DC, 2005, U.S. Department of Health and Human Services. Retrieved April 18, 2006, from http://bhpr.hrsa.gov/healthworkforce/reports/rnpopulation/preliminaryfindings.htm.

TABLE **1-2**	Comparison of Salary, Age, and Educational Levels of Nurses—2000 to 2004	
Factor	**2000**	**2004**
Average salary	$46,782	$57,784
Average age	45.2	46.8
Educational degrees		
• Diploma	23%	14.6%
• Associate's degree (2 year)	34.3%	33.7%
• Bachelor's degree (4 year)	32.7%	34.2%
• Master's or Doctoral degree	10%	13.0%

Data from Health Resources and Services Administration: *Preliminary findings: 2004 National sample survey of registered nurses,* Washington, DC, 2006 U.S. Department of Health and Human Services. Retrieved April 18, 2006, from http://bhpr.hrsa.gov/healthworkforce/reports/rnpopulation/preliminaryfindings.htm.

rather to support their countries in improving the conditions so the nurses do not need, or want to leave. The Philippines is where 50% of foreign-born nurses come from, followed by 20% from Canada, 8.4% from the United Kingdom, 2.3% from Nigeria, 1.5% from India, and 1.2% from Hong Kong (HRSA 2006).

You can see in Table 1-2 that nurses are becoming more educated. Overall the trend is toward more education to fill the growing need for nurses who can manage increasingly complex patients and health needs. Table 1-2 shows a comparison of salary, age, and educational levels of nurses between the years 2000 and 2004. The 2004 statistics are from the federal government. These were released in 2006. They are updated every 4 years. The next statistics will be for 2008 and will be released in 2010. To find updated information, go to http://bhpr.hrsa.gov.

HEALTH CARE IS CHANGING

Health care costs have grown outrageously. In an attempt to bring them down, providing care for less money has become an important issue. As a result, systems of delivering health care have evolved. You've probably heard of managed care or health maintenance organizations (HMOs) and preferred providers (PPOs). These systems are designed to provide health care to people for less money by managing their patients. Keeping people healthy is one goal; another is minimizing hospital stays when they are sick. Hospitals and health care plans are hiring "hospitalists" (i.e., doctors or nurse practitioners whose job it is to manage patient care in the hospital). Their purpose is to reduce expensive and unnecessary tests and to discharge patients as soon as they are ready to go home.

Hospitals are expensive places to provide health care because they require a large staff and expensive equipment. That's one reason why so many surgeries and procedures that used to require several days in the hospital are being done in 1 day through outpatient clinics. Examples include cataract surgery for the eyes and orthopedic procedures such as knee surgery. Having your gallbladder removed used to mean a week or more in the hospital. Now, because of new technology, it can be done safely in 1 day for a lot less money.

Nursing research is contributing to finding ways to provide quality health care for less cost. This research supplies evidence for making important health care decisions, which in turn results in better care for patients. In many cases, evidence-based practice is replacing old ways of doing things—ways that were expensive and not necessarily better for the patients.

One important advance, health promotion and disease prevention, is something nurses have been working on for over 100 years. If we can help people improve their health, there will be fewer illnesses requiring expensive hospitalization. For example, helping people quit smoking or eat a nutritious diet can have immense effects on health in terms of lung and heart disease, prenatal health, and many other conditions. Nurses want to save money, but nursing's number one concern is that people lead healthy lives and receive the best health care.

In a dramatic shift from the past, health care is moving away from treating illnesses after they occur and instead turning toward health and wellness. Nursing has always focused on health promotion and disease prevention. As far back as 1889, Florence Nightingale herself predicted this turn toward wellness. She said that by the year 2000 hospitals would be obsolete because nurses would be working to keep people well. Although this prediction has not come to pass, she was right that nurses would be working hard to keep people healthy.

Again, it is just common sense. Why not have a nurse managing people who have or are at risk for disease by teaching, counseling, assessing, and coordinating their care? It costs much less for a nurse to help a patient with heart failure, diabetes, or asthma to stay healthy than to wait for that patient to get sick enough to go to the ED and wind up in the hospital.

There will continue to be a need for hospitals for the critically ill—nurses will continue to work in emergency, intensive care, surgery, oncology, and psychiatric units just as they do now. But the main focus of health care will be on prevention and management of diseases in the home, the community, and internationally. This is precisely what the philosophy of the nursing profession is all about.

The following sections describe some of the population trends affecting health care today. Nurses are responding to these trends by expanding their roles and by revising nursing school curriculums to teach students what they will need to know to be effective nurses in the 21st century.

People Are Living Longer

The number of older people, called an *aging population*, is increasing. If you're in high school or college, your parents are probably baby boomers, and they will be making up this segment of the population. As more advances are made in technology and treatment of diseases, people are living longer. As a result, we will see more chronic illnesses such as heart disease and diabetes. People will want to live in their own homes as long as possible and remain active (this is especially going to be true of the baby boomers who take part in activities such as skiing, traveling, and kayaking). Nurses have always been experts on managing chronic illnesses—helping people to stay fit and healthy while living in their own homes—so this trend has a positive effect on nursing jobs.

Everything Costs Too Much, and We Don't Always Like It

Everyone has heard about the health care crises—rising costs and the desperate need to reduce them coupled with a general dissatisfaction with health care services. In addition, the Centers for Disease Control (National Center for Health Statistics, U.S. 2006 with Chartbook on Trends in the Health of Americans) reports health in the U.S. is not as good as most other developed countries. Life expectancy is a major health indicator. The U.S. is number 29 on a list of 30 nations for life expectancy!

Reforming health care, reducing costs, and improving access and quality remain hot social and legislative issues. Study after study shows that the number one concern of RNs is quality of care. Studies also show that RNs in hospitals improve patient outcomes by decreasing complications and death. As insurers and providers alike work to improve customer satisfaction, nurses will be called on to work in quality management, outcomes research, and public relations.

People Want Help Being Healthy

Overall we are seeing a change in health care from just treating disease and illness after they happen to trying to prevent them. The focus is more on keeping people well; and, although this is driven by a need to reduce money spent on health care, it is a positive shift in the way we run our health care system. As I just discussed, nurses have worked in health promotion and disease prevention for over 100 years. Many nurses today work in preventive programs such as nutrition, exercise, and weight management.

People Are Demanding More Information

Gone are the days when people simply did what the doctor ordered. We all want to know about the medications we take and about any tests we need. Nurses have always been the ones to inform people and help them make decisions. This trend is good for everyone, including the nursing profession. People need to be informed so they can take responsibility for their health. The Internet is full of health information, which creates another nursing role: helping people discern biased and poor information from quality evidence-based practice information. This nursing role is called informatics nursing.

So Many People; So Little Health Care

Many people, especially women and children, have no health insurance. This is a big problem. Often this is because they don't have any money. Nurses have taken political action to change laws and make policies to help people get health care. Nurses have increased the number of children in our country who are immunized against childhood diseases, advocated for children and others living in poverty, and supported safety issues such as gun control. This kind of work is part of nursing's history. Nurses started the first public health centers and homes for the poor, called *settlement houses*.

Access to health care is a huge issue, and you could go into nursing just to work on that problem alone! After all, what's the use of having a good health care system if only some of the people get to use it? This trend has a negative impact not only on nursing, but on everyone else. When families without insurance get sick, they may not be able to work. If they have to go on public assistance, we pay more as taxpayers than if their employers or the government paid their insurance benefits. Finally, families and individuals under stress are much more prone to illness and injury.

CHANGES IN HEALTH CARE AND BECOMING A NURSE

Changes in the health care system and health care professions will affect you as you choose to become a nurse, go to nursing school, and later when you work as a nurse.

Probably the most significant of these changes is the nursing shortage. There is a nursing shortage in the United States and around the world. You've heard of supply and demand in relation to the market. Supply and demand applies to nurses too.

The nursing shortage is a problem of both supply and demand. Four supply factors contribute to the shortage (Janiszewski G., 2003).*

Reasons for the Nursing Supply Shortage

Nurses Are Getting Older
The average age of an RN is about **47** years old. Between 2005 and 2010 many nurses will be retiring. Those leaving the workforce will be the most experienced nurses, leaving the health care system with too few and less experienced nurses. Remember that the aging workforce includes nurse educators. There is currently a shortage of nursing faculty that is expected to get worse.

Not Enough Students Are Enrolling in Nursing Schools
Job vacancies increase when there is a shortage of nurses to fill them. When fewer students enroll in and graduate from nursing school, the shortage increases. One reason fewer women students are enrolling in nursing school is that they have many more career options than there used to be. In the past, most college-educated women became nurses or teachers. Students today have many choices. On a positive note, with changes in people's ideas of what kinds of careers are acceptable, more men are entering nursing than ever before.

But, another, and perhaps bigger reason for a decrease in enrollment, is a lack of faculty to teach students. Nursing schools simply cannot meet the demand and many qualified applicants are turned away because there are not enough faculty to teach them. Along with a shortage of nurses is a shortage of faculty—a vicious circle that takes political will to end.

The Workplace and Job Satisfaction
The health care system has changed. To reduce costs, the amount of time a patient is in the hospital has decreased. In the past, with longer hospital stays, by the time a patient went home, he or she was more independent. How does this affect job satisfaction? Nurses used to the old system liked having lots of time to care for each patient. When patients are sicker and caseloads are heavier, nurses have less time to spend with each one. Now nurses need to be very efficient and work tirelessly with hospital leaders to make sure the quality of patient care is good.

The Poor Image of Nursing
Nursing is not always seen as a high status job. Surveys of high school students show that students may not consider a nursing career because they think nurses don't get enough respect or money. However, the same students are drawn to nursing because they want to help people. National surveys have shown that the public trusts nurses above doctors, lawyers, or any other professional.

Despite this public trust, the overall image persists that nurses are the doctor's assistants. In fact, nurses act under their own license. This means nurses are entirely responsible for their actions. Nurses are often the first line of contact, and consistently have contact with patients.

Finally, there is confusion about whether nursing is a profession or an occupation. Is nursing the same as being an electrician, or is it the same as being a lawyer or a doctor? An electrician has an occupation. Someone who practices law or medicine is a professional.

---

*Janiszewski G, Goodin H: The nursing shortage in the United States of America: an integrative review of the literature, *J Adv Nurs* 43(4): 335-343, 2003.

One reason it is difficult to view nurses as professionals is that they can have varying amounts of education. When an RN can have a diploma from a hospital, an associate's degree from a community college, or a bachelor's degree from a university, it is difficult to judge just how educated that RN is. We know that professions such as law or medicine require a lot of education; that is part of how we judge them to be professions. Nursing is more confusing. If it takes only 2 years to become an RN, people may think that nurses are not educated enough to be considered professionals. Students who desire a high level of intellectual challenge may pass up nursing. Of course, nurses are professionals, whether they have an associate's degree from a community college or a bachelor's degree from a university. A nurse is independent and responsible for her or his actions (see Chapter 5 for more on nursing education levels).

Reasons for the Increasing Demand for Nurses

People Are Living Longer
Because people are living longer, more and more people have chronic health problems. Think about what kinds of health concerns older people have. High blood pressure, diabetes, and arthritis are just a few. People can live very well with these problems, but the number of people with them is increasing very quickly. We have and will continue to have an increasing number of older people in the U.S. population. Nurses are needed to manage these illnesses, to teach people how to live with them, and to help people with prevention.

Increased Diversity in the U.S. Population
It is estimated that by 2050 over 50% of the population in the U.S. will be non-Caucasian. Caucasian, non-Hispanic people are now in the majority, except in some states. This is changing rapidly, and health care professions are not keeping up with the changes. Nursing is the most ethnically diverse health profession, but that isn't saying much. Nursing is still about 86% Caucasian, non-Hispanic. Nursing and other health professions definitely do not reflect the makeup of the U.S. population. It is necessary to have health providers from all ethnic groups and cultures.

People in Hospitals Need More Nursing Care
People in hospitals are sicker. Why is that? At one time people stayed in the hospital for a longer time for any given problem. For instance, when I first became a nurse, a patient who had open-heart surgery stayed about a week. By the end of that week the patient was doing pretty well and didn't need as much care. Therefore I could care for more patients because no one patient required intensive care. Now a person having open-heart surgery goes home in a few days. During the time spent in the hospital, the patient is less able to do anything for himself or herself. The term used for this is *acuity*. Acuity reflects how much care patients need. The greater the acuity, the more care they need. Patients in hospitals are sicker so the acuity is higher. A nurse cannot safely care for as many patients. In other words, the higher the acuity, the fewer patients any one nurse can care for. Therefore more nurses are needed. The demand has gone up. One reason the acuity has increased is that patients are discharged sooner to save money.

Increased Opportunities for Nurses Outside Hospitals
Nurses are more in demand than ever. They are working for pharmaceutical companies and other technology-related companies. The need for community health and public health nurses has also increased.

Increased Demand for Faculty as We Try to Recruit and Graduate More Nurses

The average age of a nurse educator is 51 years old—not too far from retirement. As noted above, since the demand for nurses is growing, we need more nurse educators to educate them!

Four Solutions to the Nursing Shortage

1. Increase recruitment of students (especially students of color and men) into nursing. Improving the image and understanding of nursing is a way to attract people into the profession.
2. Keep those in nursing. This is also called retention. Improving the conditions in the workplace is seen as one way to retain nurses. Figure 1-1 illustrates the Nurses Bill of Rights.
3. Government can help the nursing shortage by continuing to fund scholarships, research into workforce issues, and colleges and universities. Educating a nurse costs a school a lot more per student than most other degrees. Nursing schools need federal assistance to maintain or increase enrollment. Of course, nursing faculty are also needed to teach students. If we increase the number of students to meet the demand for more nurses, we have to have more faculty.
4. Increase nursing salaries to attract more qualified young people into the profession.

CONCERNS ABOUT CHANGES IN HEALTH CARE

Professional nurses are deeply concerned with the nursing shortage, but there are other issues that the American Nurses Association and other specialty nursing groups are working on. One of these is the problem of the uninsured. Forty-four million people, or 15.2% of the U.S. population, including children, do not have access to health care because of lack of insurance. Many nurses think that affordable, safe, and effective health care is a human right and that it shouldn't be withheld because of economic or other considerations. You can find out more about these by going to the American Nurses Association website and looking at the Agenda for the Future (http://nursingworld.org/naf/) and the Health Care Agenda (http://nursingworld.org/member/practice/).

But enough politics for now—the purpose of this book is to help you understand what a nurse is, what it takes to be a nurse, if you want to become one, and if so, how to go about it. So let's get going. No blood, no guts, but lots of glory.

The American Nurses Association's

Bill of Rights
for Registered Nurses

Registered nurses promote and restore health, prevent illness and protect the people entrusted to their care. They work to alleviate the suffering experienced by individuals, families, groups and communities. In so doing, nurses provide services that maintain respect for human dignity and embrace the uniqueness of each patient and the nature of his or her health problems, without restriction with regard to social or economic status. To maximize the contributions nurses make to society, it is necessary to protect the dignity and autonomy of nurses in the workplace. To that end, the following rights must be afforded:

I. Nurses have the right to practice in a manner that fulfills their obligations to society and to those who receive nursing care.

II. Nurses have the right to practice in environments that allow them to act in accordance with professional standards and legally authorized scopes of practice.

III. Nurses have the right to a work environment that supports and facilitates ethical practice, in accordance with the Code of Ethics for Nurses and its interpretive statements.

IV. Nurses have the right to freely and openly advocate for themselves and their patients, without fear of retribution.

V. Nurses have the right to fair compensation for their work, consistent with their knowledge, experience and professional responsibilities.

VI. Nurses have the right to a work environment that is safe for themselves and their patients.

VII. Nurses have the right to negotiate the conditions of their employment, either as individuals or collectively, in all practice settings.

AMERICAN NURSES ASSOCIATION • 600 MARYLAND AVENUE, SW, SUITE 100 WEST • WASHINGTON, DC 20024
NURSINGWORLD.ORG

Adopted by ANA Board of Directors: June 26, 2001   © Copyright 2001, American Nurses Association

FIGURE **1-1**
Bill of Rights for registered nurses. From American Nurses Association: The American Nurses Association's Bill of Rights for Registered Nurses, Washington, DC, 2001, Author.

Chapter

2

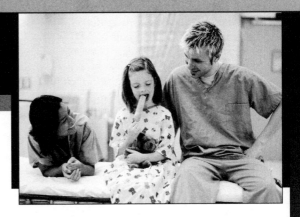

Tell Someone Who Cares

"Strength, Commitment, Compassion" was the motto for the 2006 National Nurses' Week. "Nurses have the courage to care" was one of my favorite mottos from the 1997 National Nurses' Week and something people say over and over about nurses. My friend's 15-year-old daughter Alisha told me, "Someone who is going to be a nurse has to be a caring person." She's right, but what does it mean to care?

Compassion, knowledge, honesty, and commitment are components of caring, according to nursing theory, which states that caring is "the essence" of nursing practice. You probably have your own ideas. You care about a friend, you care about how you look and feel, you care for a pet, you care about your family. You could say caring means that you have good feelings for someone or something, that you want him or her to do well, and that you may even love the person or thing (e.g., a pet).

Here's what a group of senior nursing students had to say about caring:
"Caring means giving close attention."
"Giving of yourself."
"To be helpful and nurturing."
"Caring is being concerned."
"Caring is the same as meeting needs."

Caring is thinking about what you would want for yourself or for your family and then, as many nurses do, using that to guide you in your work, even when you're under pressure. The workload is heavy, you're tired, and there's too much to do in too little time, but as a nurse you will be thinking, "What would I want for this patient if he or she were my mother, my child, or myself?"

For example, when Sharon was a new nurse working in a small hospital, she took care of a young first-time mother and her husband. It was time for the woman to deliver, but the baby had died before birth. The woman still had to go through labor to deliver the baby. Sharon worked overtime into the next shift caring for this family and helping them physically and emotionally through a very painful experience. She said, "I just kept thinking about what I would want and need if I were the one going through that. When I got so tired and felt overwhelmed with the tragedy, this kept me going."

Caring is a nursing value. Values guide your work and your life; they provide a foundation for your actions. Other nursing values include compassion, advocacy, respect for the rights and beliefs of others, justice, knowledge, and honesty. Caring is manifest in all sorts of ways, not just between a nurse and patient or family. Carol Bonnono, RN, worked as an Emergency Department (ED) nurse in Oregon and cared enough about accident victims of drunk drivers that she went to her state governor about it. Until the time Carol took action, because of patient privacy rights, ED nurses were not permitted to report patients with alcohol levels above 0.15% to the police. She said:

> As an ED nurse, I was outraged when I learned this. I strongly believe that ED personnel should not only be allowed but also required to inform law officers of patients whose blood alcohol level exceeds legal limits. I was treating the same people week after week for injuries sustained in motor vehicle accidents they caused by driving while intoxicated, and I could do nothing but help stitch them up and send them back out on the road.

Oregon now has a law that changed reporting requirements, and in the first year, there was a 1% reduction in alcohol-related fatalities. On a national level, Oregon congresswoman Elizabeth Furse introduced a bill, House Resolution 1982, which she calls the "Carol Bonnono Bill." Carol, who considers herself a patient advocate like all other nurses, turned her frustration and anger into action motivated by her caring.

WHO CARES WHO CURES?

Do doctors only cure illness and nurses only care for the people who are ill? The main differences between doctors and nurses are the principles and goals guiding their work. A nurse's primary mission is to care for people before, during, or after episodes of illness. A doctor's is to diagnose and cure illnesses. These basic premises form the foundation of each profession's practice, but they do not limit it. For instance, nurses often diagnose and cure illnesses, whereas doctors care for and comfort their patients. This role overlap leads to confusion about the distinct individuality of the two professions. The American Nurses Association defines nursing in the Scope and Standards of Practice: "Nursing is the protection, promotion, and optimization of health and abilities, prevention of illness and injury, alleviation of suffering through the diagnosis and treatment of human response, and advocacy in the care of individuals, families, communities and populations."

Nurses do many things to help people get over an illness. Nurse practitioners can diagnose health problems and prescribe medications to treat those problems. For instance, Cherrie, a nationally certified family nurse practitioner with a master's degree in nursing, has prescription authority in the state of Washington. (This authorization to prescribe drugs varies from state to state.) She has worked in an office with a family doctor, has had her own patients, has diagnosed their problems, and has prescribed treatments. When she needs help, she talks with the doctor, consults with a specialist, or refers the patient to one.

Curing is easier to describe than caring (which is one very good reason why nursing is hard to define). Think of a time when you felt cared for or when you cared for someone else. Would it be hard to describe that experience? A student in one of my classes, Nancy, described caring by telling a story about a patient to whom she was assigned. She was going in to assess him after he had a CT scan to look for lung cancer. Although he appeared to be resting quietly in bed, she only had to take one look at him to know how frightened he was:

> I looked into his eyes and saw fear—fear as plain as day. He was absolutely petrified. So I sat down next to him, took his hand, and asked him how he was. He began to cry. I continued to hold his hand, and he cried for a while. He told me that I was the first person that day to pay any attention to him.

The man had been in the hospital all day getting tests and interacting with doctors, technicians, hospital personnel, and other nurses. At the end of the day, he felt that Nancy was the first to pay attention to him as a person and not just as a case. Nancy understood that he was vulnerable and in a frightening situation. By letting him express his fear, she cared for him in a way that no one else did, and with what we know today about mind-body interactions, caring can be part of the cure.

Another nursing student, Karen, described caring as follows:

> When my grandfather was in the hospital, the nurses were the ones who were there all the time. They were interested in us and how we felt. When he went home, they made sure we had all the information we needed. The doctors, on the other hand, came in and out of the room. They checked Grandpa briefly and left. The nurses were the most important to us.

Alisha, mentioned previously, experienced caring after an injury in ballet class:

> When I went to the Emergency Department with a twisted ankle, the nurse was very nice. He talked to me and told me everything he was doing. He taught me how to take care of my ankle. He was good.

Another way to think about caring is to think about comfort. Research has shown that making patients comfortable is essential to good nursing care. Researcher Katherine Kolcaba, RN, PhD put it this way:

> We have long recognized that comfortable patients heal faster, cope better, become rehabilitated more thoroughly, or die more peacefully than do the uncomfortable. Patient comfort is the essence of nursing and contributes to patients' quality of life.

WHO'S WHO IN THE HEALTH CARE ZOO?

Health care is a term that covers everything from nursing to medicine to homeopathy. To better understand nursing you have to understand the place of different professions within the health care system. Health care professionals do all sorts of things to help people improve their health, whether they are sick or not. Think of going for a sports physical. You're not sick, but you need to be checked to make sure it is safe for you to play sports.

On the other hand, you may be very sick with a bacterial infection in your throat. In this case, you get health care that hopefully will cure your sickness. Or you may go to a clinic to check for sexually transmitted diseases. It's a routine visit, and you may not be sick at all. You will receive information and have your questions answered by experts in that field. If you have a disease, you will receive treatment. These types of examinations, education, and treatment can be provided by nurses or doctors.

Nurses can do all the things listed above: giving sports physicals, educating patients, treating infections, and answering questions. Doctors do too. The key point is that nursing and medicine are different professions with different focuses. Doctors diagnose and treat diseases; nurses promote health and educate and care for families. Think of a physical therapist, a dentist, an acupuncturist, a registered dietitian, and a social worker. These people are all in health care professions. But their jobs are all different.

More confusing are the differences between registered nurses (RNs), licensed practical nurses (LPNs), and physician's assistants (PAs). LPNs have 1-2 years of training, most often work in hospitals and nursing homes, and perform less complicated work than RNs. PAs are commonly confused with nurse practitioners. Nurse practitioners (RNs who have obtained a graduate degree in nursing) usually practice under their state's nursing board. PAs usually, but not always, have previous health care experience (e.g., as a medic in the military) and then attend a program that is 1 to 2 years in length. PAs work under the physician's license.

Nurses receive an extraordinary education that gives them the unique and broad view needed to treat the whole person (this is also referred to as holistic healing). While studying nursing in college, you will take classes in the humanities such as education, multicultural studies, and fine arts, in addition to sciences such as pathophysiology and pharmacology. Nurses also need political knowledge to work on making changes that will improve health care services; courses such as psychology and history to help them work with diverse populations; and sociology to help solve family and other social problems such as domestic violence and meeting the unique needs of elders or teenagers.

Again, this is why it is hard to describe nursing—there is so much to it—and at the same time this is why nursing has so many fascinating opportunities. At this point, you should be starting to see that nursing is not what you thought or perhaps that it includes more than you thought. Nursing is not just a chance to get a quick job in a hospital helping people feel better. It is about a commitment to knowledge and, as a professional, to learning whatever you need to care for and cure people.

A WOMAN'S WORK IS NEVER DONE: BUT WHO CARES!

Before Florence Nightingale appeared on the scene in the mid-19th century, women were responsible for taking care of sick family members in the home. This was because hospitals used to be terribly unsanitary places where patients, three or four to a bed, went to die rather than to be healed. Knowledge about many diseases, especially infectious diseases, was lacking. Even farther back in history most nurses in European societies were men affiliated with religious or military orders.

Florence Nightingale, the most famous nurse in history, although not the most important, used her talent and knowledge acquired in the Crimean War to reform hospitals. Some of her most important work had to do with the design and management of hospitals based on her theory that, in a proper environment, nature could heal. Her theory holds true today. Cleanliness, fresh air, and good nutrition are things that nurses use today to promote health and prevent illness. Another important nurse who worked with Nightingale is less known. Mary Seacole, a nurse from Jamaica, also served in the Crimea. Her portrait hangs in the National Portrait Gallery in London. Other nurses of color include abolitionists Sojourner Truth and Harriet Tubman, Civil War nurse Susie Taylor, and Spanish-American War nurse Namahyoke Sockum.

Florence Nightingale is most often portrayed as an angel of mercy, and she has been remembered for this image rather than for her work as a nurse. Nightingale was born into a rich, educated English family, received an excellent education, and traveled extensively. Her biggest problem was that she wanted to do meaningful work. Women of her day, especially upper-class women, did not work outside the home. If they did, it was usually out of necessity—in other words, because they were poor. As a wealthy, educated woman, it was expected that Florence would marry.

She had to choose between doing what her family wanted and becoming a nurse. Today this would not be such a difficult decision. But for her it meant a choice between giving up what she wanted and being alienated from and possibly disowned by her family. Florence left her family to become a nurse and for many years had no contact with her mother or sister. Her writing shows how painful this was for her, but she considered her work important enough to sacrifice this contact.

In 1854, Nightingale was asked by the British government to go to the Crimea, where England was at war. She was excited about this opportunity but probably had no idea what she was getting into. She was shocked and horrified by the conditions in which she found both the injured and the healthy soldiers living. There was no sanitation, raw sewage water was used in cooking, and drinking water was contaminated by animal carcasses that lay in the streams.

She organized and restructured the camps and, in so doing, saved the lives of thousands. Late at night, she wrote letters to the government that resulted in radical changes, and she is credited with being the person most effective in British history in improving the status and treatment of the British soldier.

Nightingale also kept detailed records of what happened during her time in the Crimea. She recorded the number of men who lived and died and the number and types of their injuries. As such, she became the first biostatistician (someone who records statistics on humans). After her outstanding work in the Crimea, she was a worldwide heroine. Everyone knew her name, just as they do today.

Eventually she talked to her family again, but she never married. In fact, nurses, like teachers, by law could not marry because having children and making a living by taking care of people were not viewed as being compatible. Furthermore, there were no male nurses—you had to be a woman to be a nurse. So nursing was literally and legally women's work and that fact has had a profound impact on the profession, in terms of both salary and image.

Joe, who started out as a medic in Vietnam, told me how he thought it affected his money-making ability:

> I am very aware of nursing as woman's work and that it is thought of that way. Women always take care of people, especially sick people. They are expected to do it. It is supposed to come naturally. That's why we don't get paid as much for what we do.

Theo Alkin, RN, working in a large ED, pointed out similarly how it affects image:

> Because nurses are women, we are expected to do all the things we do. It is supposed to come naturally. People don't think as highly about what we do. We just do it."

What this means to you as a potential nurse is that you'll inherit some problems. It isn't news that women make less money than men. Lower pay is generally connected to work that involves caring for others such as nursing and teaching. Ask yourself this question: Why do doctors generally have more status or prestige than nurses?

An obvious answer would be that traditionally nurses are women and doctors are men. Or you could say it is because society values the type of work doctors do, curing, over what nurses do, caring. Take a look at a magazine or newspaper article about health care and you'll see that doctors are the main feature. Likewise, when I see a preview of a show on TV that's going to be about health care, I know that it will be about doctors, and 99% of the time I'm right. One study showed that literature on health policy and issues rarely mentions nurses, despite the fact that nurses make up the largest group of health care providers.

Another answer to this question is that doctors have more responsibility than nurses. But how do you define responsibility? Does a teacher who spends the entire day, day after day, with a young child developing a lifetime of learning have as much responsibility as a doctor who sees that same child for 5 minutes about an earache? Does a nurse who manages the medications and care of 20 patients have less responsibility than a doctor who performs the removal of a gallbladder? As a society, we say that the doctor has more responsibility and therefore more value.

Responsibility and value are defined by individuals and by the culture of the dominant society. Some of these definitions are changing, though (and if I have anything to do with it, they will). Health promotion and disease prevention, professional responsibilities of nursing, are gaining importance. Likewise, RNs are beginning to be recognized for this important aspect of their work. But this recognition has largely been our own doing. Instead of meekly waiting for someone to come along and notice us, we're out on the street corners shouting our own praise and in research laboratories crunching numbers to statistically show the value of our work.

In nursing a high level of technical and clinical skills combine with caring skills to provide comfort and save lives. Pat, a neonatal flight nurse, demonstrated this late one night as she transported a critical newborn via helicopter from a small hospital to a larger medical center:

One night we transported a ventilator-dependent baby with a massive pulmonary hemorrhage. The baby was in critical condition, so we also brought her mother on board. I wanted the mother to see that I was doing all I could for her baby—not everyone will do that, but that is important to me. Coming back to the hospital, the weather was really crappy. The rain and wind were so strong that we were blown around like rag dolls. The pilot couldn't even make out the horizon. All the lights on board the helicopter had to be turned off so the pilot could navigate by street and car lights below. The only light we had to work with was from the monitor, and even that had to be screened from the pilot.

Suddenly I noticed on the monitor that the baby's oxygen was dropping quickly. I got out my flashlight and began searching for clues. Immediately I could see that the baby was bleeding from her mouth so badly that it caused the security tape on the breathing tube to come loose. The tube had slipped out of the baby's mouth. She quickly became symptomatic; her blood pressure dropped and heart rate went way up. In these kinds of situations we flight nurses look at a monitor, see something happen, and ask ourselves, "What does this mean?" And we have to work it through very quickly and determine what to do and then do it fast.

Here we were, up in the air with no lights, and the only light I had was this little flashlight that I held in my mouth while I went to work. The baby was lying on her side in the Isolette, bleeding profusely from the mouth. On top of that, the mother was on board, so we really had no room to move around. The baby's mother realized something had gone wrong, but she really didn't know what was happening. She sat in her jump seat with terror in her eyes and tears running down her face.

The baby needed to be reintubated (her breathing tube had to be put back in), but I couldn't see how it could be done in this predicament. Intubation is complicated under the best conditions, especially with infants. All of these thoughts ran through my head in a fraction of a second. Still, I was left with no choice. In the darkness I reached both arms into the portholes of the Isolette. With one gloved finger, I blindly lifted up the epiglottis (at the back of the baby's throat). With the other hand, I guided a new tube into the airway. It worked, and immediately the vital signs stabilized.

We got to the hospital, and the baby and mother eventually went home. The mother was exceptionally grateful that I had the skills to handle that crisis and that she could be there while I cared for her baby.

WE CARE TOO: MEN IN NURSING

In my graduate nursing research class, a student, Paul, had two earrings, drove a motorcycle, and worked in a hospital ED. He was 26 years old and had just gotten married. As the semester progressed, I asked him why he had become a nurse.

"My mother wanted me to," he joked. "She's a nurse, but when I was thinking about what to do after high school, nursing seemed a good option. I liked science and I was interested in health. I thought it would be a good job to learn in, and one that I could keep learning in."

One day in class we talked about conflict in the workplace. One of the students described her attempts to persuade hospital administrators that more nurses were needed on her unit to safely take care of patients. The administrators responded, "We don't have the money. Make do with what you have." The student was extremely frustrated by the interaction, and, because she didn't feel secure in further discussion, much less confrontation, she dropped the subject.

Paul listened carefully and said, "That's when you need the support of other nurses: to make your point with a unified voice. If people don't like it, don't act rude or anything, but don't back down."

I liked that. This sums up a great deal of what nursing is about today. Nurses have to be able to work together for change in an environment that does not always favor what the nurses think. Nurses think first about quality of care. To work in health care today, one needs skill and the ability to negotiate and come to agreeable compromises. Paul was able to pinpoint a solution.

Men in Nursing Survey

In 2004, 498 men in nursing took a survey to determine why they thought there were so few men in their chosen profession. Survey questions looked at challenges men face in nursing, reasons men are not attracted to nursing, and misperceptions about men in nursing.

Many of the survey respondents said that choosing a career in nursing was the best decision they had ever made, whereas others said they would choose a different career. Some men thought that the name of the profession would have to change because the title *nurse* was sexist. An excerpt from the website report of the survey (www.hodes.com/industries/healthcare/resources/research/meninnursingsurvey.asp), conducted by the Bernard Hodes Group (an employment advertising agency), states the following:

Nursing is much more than just holding someone's hand. It is mathematics, no less than construction. It is science, no less than a chemist. It is task management, no less than a CEO. It is research, no less than a detective. It is hard work, no less than manual labor. It is giving, caring and guidance, no less than any advisor. It is multitasking, no less than a foreman. It is nurturing strengths and working with the weaknesses, no less than a chaplain. It is helping others be all they can be, just like the ad for the Army. It is accepting that women have strengths, as well as nurturing skills. It is accepting that men have compassion, as well as caring skills.

Nurses do things that both men and women can do. There is nothing about nursing, except our image of it, that makes it necessary to be a woman. Caring, communicating, making decisions, working for health—these are all things both men and women can do.

As stated in Chapter 1, only 5.7% of all nurses are men, but that is changing as the number of men going to nursing school increases. There are more men going into nursing; 12% to 13% of nursing school graduates are men (NLN, 2006).

Why is this? Nursing offers options, challenges, and rewards to both men and women. As our society becomes less focused on outmoded gender roles, everyone's options for work increases. Just as you see women working in careers traditionally held by men, men are working in careers traditionally held by women. Stereotypes are breaking down slowly, but they are breaking down. The days when it was a requirement to be a woman in order to become a nurse have disappeared.

Men do face problems in nursing, though; and the one most frequently mentioned is "role strain" or pressures related to working in a traditionally female profession. Many men choose to work in emergency or psychiatric departments or as nurse anesthetists, which are areas some perceive to be less dominated by women. However, Christine Williams, a University of Texas sociologist, studied men in women's professions and found that men don't get harassed as much as women do for stepping across the gender line; they are promoted faster, and it's more likely men will feel welcomed.

Talking to men in nursing, I was curious whether they faced discrimination or assumptions about their masculinity. Did people see them as less of a man for being a nurse? None of the men I talked to had this problem. Paul said that his older brothers teased him at times, but he said they teased him about everything. He had no problems at work from either patients or other staff.

I worked with Bill in the cardiac intensive care unit, and he told me that being a man in nursing meant that some people thought you were the doctor. It's automatic to regard a man as the doctor and a woman as the nurse. He would correct them by saying, "I'm not a doctor; I'm a nurse. I'll be taking care of you and managing your care this evening." He was a favorite of everyone, patients and staff. He was funny and smart and an excellent nurse.

Another nurse, Justin, was a flight nurse. The flight service covered over 200 nautical miles and was the fourth largest in the United States. Justin, who loved flight nursing, said he became a nurse because he liked people and science and he wanted a secure job making a decent amount of money. He had a lot of autonomy in his work; when the team went on a flight, he was in charge of the patient's care. There were no doctors on board or on the radio. Justin decided what to do and how to do it. He had worked hard to get to this point in his career, but he said it had been worth it, and "I've had the best job in the world."

Mike was a BSN student I met in a community health clinical course I taught. He was about 28 years old and had originally wanted to become a doctor. He went to a good university and graduated with a degree and a high GPA. He applied to medical school for several years but was never accepted. While volunteering in a hospital ED, he had ample opportunity to observe the different members of the health care team. During that time he noticed that nurses had a great deal of independence; did most of the patient teaching and work with families; acted as the go-between with doctors, pharmacists, social workers, and law enforcement; and, best of all, were real patient advocates. Now, as Mike was just about to graduate from nursing school, I asked him if he had any regrets. He said, "Absolutely not!" He now knew that nursing was a better profession for him, and he was actually glad he had never been accepted into medical school.

In Chapter 1 I talked about considering a nursing career for the wrong reasons. Another way to look at this is: "Are you *not* considering nursing for the wrong reasons?" A survey of college males suggested that, if men were given more information about nursing, they would consider it as a career. The primary reason men stay away from nursing is social; as long as nursing is thought of as mainly a women's profession, participation by men will continue to be small. If you are a man and the reason you are not thinking much about nursing is that you think it is a career for women, think again. Don't let your view of gender limit you to a certain type of work. Think about what you want to do and then look at what nursing has to offer in terms of challenges and rewards. Many women have broken into fields previously populated only by men. If women can do it, men can, too.

CARING MEANS MANY THINGS

Nurses tell stories about their work that show how caring affects their patients. Caring means many things: taking time to listen, advocating for those in need, being open-minded, and making pain relief a priority. Liz, a home health care nurse, spoke about helping a woman with severe postpartum depression. Her story details how caring involves advocating and being open-minded:

> She was so depressed that she was talking about leaving her family—her husband and her four children (one an infant). It was really a bad situation. She didn't think she was a good parent or that she was worth anything. I got in touch with her husband and made sure he understood the severity of her depression. I also spoke to her doctor and got her in to see a counselor. Later, when she recovered, she said to me many times, "I really appreciate you because you didn't think of me as a crazy person; you just thought of me as a normal person who was having a hard time. I don't know what would have happened without you."

Elthea has been a nurse for 24 years. She is soft-spoken and appears shy when she talks. She once worked in the ED of a large regional hospital and trauma center and spoke about how relieving pain is an important aspect of caring:

> I had a patient who came to the ED with very painful kidney stones. I worked with her and told the doctor and nurses, "You know, we have to get her an IVP (a test for kidney stones), but it needs to wait until I get her pain under control." That's just routine for me; that's how I do things. I think it's a nice thing to be able to have your pain relieved before you have x-rays. This is just part of my practice—to relieve someone's pain before the person has to go and have worse pain.
>   The next day she sent me flowers. It really made me feel good. I thought, wow, it's really nice that this person would send me this kind of thing. It doesn't happen often; that's why I was so surprised.

With the care of the patient always their first priority, some nurses may stretch a hospital rule. Julie, working with a young man with terminal cancer, was mainly concerned for his comfort and needs as he was about to die:

> He was going to die soon, and he so badly wanted to see his little puppy again, so we snuck his puppy into his room for him. If you were really rigid and went strictly by the books, that kind of thing wouldn't be done. But, to me, not to listen to something that was so important to him when he was dying was wrong, too. It really didn't make any difference at all in the grand scheme of things if the puppy came into the hospital. But it made a lot of difference to him, so we did it; and it made him smile for the first time in a long time. It was well worth it.

Tell someone who cares? Tell a nurse. Nursing has a century of caring behind it. Caring is like the foundation of a house; it holds all that is built on it and shapes and secures the house. Caring is nursing's ground—its roots. It holds the profession in place and guides the work of nurses as individually they build their careers and, as a group, their profession.

Chapter

3

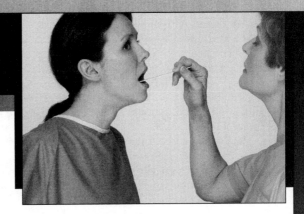

Making a Career Decision is Enough to Make Anyone Sick

Personally I never really knew what I wanted to be when I grew up, but I had many ideas. When I was very little, I wanted to be a beauty queen–movie star and then a psychologist who knew everything in the world. Later I wanted to be a part-time veterinarian, part-time plant pathologist, a horseshoer-blacksmith-artist, and then…well, the list goes on.

Nursing came to me by accident. I worked in many different jobs, but the one I enjoyed most was as a crisis counselor and assistant in a family planning clinic in Massachusetts. I liked talking to people, and I was interested in science and in health. Perhaps more important, I was at a point where I really needed to do something that would not only land me a job but give me one with a positive long-term outlook—a career.

As I thought about nursing, potentially it seemed to be the perfect combination of counselor, scientist, and health expert. Thus, even though after many years on and off in college I was only one class away from a degree in biology, I switched majors to nursing and stayed in school for 2½ more years. I even returned to school 10 years after graduating to earn my master's degree in nursing and then 2 years after that to earn my Ph.D. Being a nurse has turned out to be worth it. It has become much more to me than "a job." Nursing is intriguing, exciting, and a challenge that has taught me at least as much about myself as it has about the world around me.

GROWING UP OR THROWING UP?

As you must be well aware at this point, trying to decide on a career is not easy. The fear of making a wrong decision is as powerful as your worries about the money, time, and energy needed to reach your goals. What you do for work helps shape your self-image and, as such, is enough to make you a bit queasy. Whether the butterflies in your stomach are from fear or excitement or both, ask yourself this question, "Do I picture myself working in a service profession?" If the answer is yes, then congratulations; at least you're on the right track. Nurses, doctors, pharmacists, physical therapists, respiratory therapists, and nutritionists are all members of health professions that offer opportunities to work with and serve other people.

To help you clear your mind and get down to reality, follow the steps outlined in the following sections; they will help you answer the question: "What do all these health care professionals really do?"

Step 1: Look at Each Profession

What do people in these professions do every day? Do you see yourself doing it? I know people who hate hospitals. They say that even the smell makes them sick. Don't rule out a health career, especially nursing, for this reason. Many nurses work in clinics, universities, and people's homes. Besides, you can get used to the smell. One teenager told me that the one thing she thought she would hate about nursing was that nurses wore very ugly, thick shoes. Unsightly shoes—now there's a reason for a career choice! Not to worry, though—many nurses wear light athletic shoes or cushioned clogs.

Step 2: Make a List of Pros and Cons

If you are thinking of being a medical technician, a Pro might be that you'd work with laboratory tests, something that interests you. A Con might be that you like working with people and the medical technician field wouldn't provide much opportunity to do that or that you would want to be more flexible in the location of your work. If you wanted to be a doctor, a Pro might be that you could work and live anywhere you wanted. A Con might be that you would have to go to school for a very long time.

You might be interested in nursing because you want to help people. A Pro would be that most nurses work directly with people. A Con might be that changes in health care mean that nurses frequently deal with change—change of work locations, change of policies, or change of political views affecting nursing practice. If you don't want that, consider another health care career.

Step 3: Experience the Profession Firsthand

This is most important—find someone doing the work you are interested in and ask her to let you follow her around for several weeks, a day, or even just for a few hours (the "anything's better than nothing" approach). This is the best way to get an idea of what really goes on in any job and to find out if you are interested in that kind of work. Ask your school counselor to help you find someone, or ask a friend or parent who can help you.

• • •

Some regard health care as an opportunity to find a satisfying career; others regard it as just a job. Some think of it as both. I hope you don't go into nursing just because you need a job, although I have to admit that I do know a nurse or two who has done so. Luckily they found that they loved the work and went on for more education so that nursing could really become a career for them.

However, I would not recommend this route. Don't become a nurse just to get a job. The profession is far too demanding for that. If you first try to find out if it is what you want to do, you'll save yourself a great deal of hard, frustrating work and heartache. See if you fit one of the following scenarios or if you are a combination of several.

Ask yourself the following questions about making a nursing career decision.

A. *Are you thinking about what to do after high school to get a job quickly and with reasonable pay?*

If you are thinking of nursing, you are probably thinking of going to community college for a 2-year registered nurse (RN) program. This will be fairly inexpensive and quick. You will find a job in a hospital, perhaps in a clinic, or most likely in an extended-care facility such as a nursing home. Sound good? There are many reasons to take this option, but remember that if you want to make nursing a career and advance in the profession, you'll need a bachelor's degree in nursing.

I taught in a program for RNs returning to earn their bachelor's degree. They told me, "I wish I had done it all at once. It would have saved me a lot of time." "I need the 4-year degree to get to a higher pay scale." "I need the 4-year degree to get a promotion." Other nurses who have found a job they like—in a hospital, for example—are entirely happy with a 2-year degree. They are expert clinical nurses, they like where they are, and they plan to stay there.

B. *Are you a senior in high school who wants to get a job in health care mainly because you are interested in science?*

You're probably thinking about many different health care possibilities, including working in a medical laboratory, in respiratory therapy, as a cardiovascular technician, as a nurse, or as a doctor. Your considerations in making a career choice, if you are similar to many other students, are length and cost of schooling, eventual salary, prestige, authority, and interest in the work.

An example of a nurse with these characteristics, Jasmine, a family nurse practitioner, makes a very good salary, has autonomy and power, and loves her work.

Carlos was vice president of patient care services at a large urban hospital. In this capacity he made decisions that affected hundreds of people, garnered respect, and made more than the average hospital nursing administrator's salary of $88,000 to over $150,000 (University of California San Francisco 2006). He no longer practiced nursing in a clinical situation, he kept his license current and considered his nursing experience with patients invaluable in his executive-level job. Amile is a nurse anesthetist who earns close to the national average salary for a nurse anesthetist of $164,172 a year, (CRNA Salary Survey 2006) and works with an independent group of nurses who contract with hospitals for their services.

You can see that there are nurses who do not conform to the stereotypes; you don't have to, either. If you like science and want to work with people, nursing may be for you.

C. Are you currently going to college and not sure what to do for a career?

You want to study something that will help you find a job that will be interesting, require brainpower, offer opportunity for advancement, and give you some respect and power.

First, how good are you in the sciences? To be a nurse you'll have to enjoy or learn to enjoy them. Nursing requires daily use of science, especially an understanding of the scientific process. How a nurse thinks and acts is often based on this method of problem solving. To learn how to think like a researcher is important because you must always be asking yourself, "Why am I doing it this way?" "Is the procedure or treatment best for the patient?" "Is it best for the patient and cost-effective?" "Is this treatment evidenced-based practice?"

Second, do you want to work in health care? Obviously this is a key point in your decision making. As I've mentioned before, talk to people in the different fields and then observe what they do.

D. Are you in another job and want to do something different or more interesting?

Many nurses have had other jobs outside of health care, myself included. I worked in family planning, in a research laboratory, and on a farm, to name a few. Peggy worked identifying and cataloging plant species in the wilds of Alaska, as a fish packer, and as a mapmaker. Some of the best nurses have had previous careers. These experiences are valuable and add to your qualifications to become a nurse. (See the following section on second-career RNs.)

E. Are you majoring in premed?

A seasoned nursing adviser at a large state university told me that many of the students she sees are in the premed program. You may well ask why they were seeing her.

These premed students tell her the following reasons:

- "I want to be a doctor, but the science courses required are tougher than I thought they would be."
- "I thought I wanted to be a doctor. But now I see that I don't, because I don't want to go to school for so long."

Heidi was an excellent high school student from a small farming community where the doctor was very family-oriented. She loved science and saw herself becoming a doctor like the one in her town. She struggled with the science and math classes in college. She thought nursing might be an easier alternative and decided to look into changing majors.

Her prenursing college adviser told her that nursing was not the same as being a doctor, nor was it easier, but maybe she could still do what she loved and work in a small town. The adviser hooked Heidi up with a nurse practitioner who worked in the country. She was the only health care provider for a large farming and logging community. Heidi followed her around for a few days and discovered that this was exactly what she wanted to do. She went back to school, worked with a tutor in the science classes, and changed her major from premed to nursing. This time she did so for the right reason.

Another premed student, James Hall, worked with a physician in a small hospital between his first and second years of college. As he and the doctor went on morning rounds, James began to notice what the nurses did and soon realized that their work was more like what he wanted to do. Why? He said, "I saw that the nurses had far more contact with the patients and their families than the doctor did. The nurses spent more time educating and working on preventive care, and that was what I wanted to do." He changed his major from premed to nursing for the right reasons.

James' choice is an example of an excellent reason for changing your major. He observed that nurses were different from doctors and, by comparing the two roles, discovered that he preferred the latter.

In Chapter 1 I talked about nursing stereotypes and how much of what nurses do is unseen by the casual observer: the thinking process, decision making, evaluating, coordinating, and perhaps most important, the way RNs advocate for the good of the patient and family. Many of the stories in this book show how nurses act as advocates, but perhaps Liz's story of working in oncology shows best the importance of this unique nursing role, as she advocated for her patient dying from leukemia:

> He was in bad shape—everyone knew he was dying. His platelet count was really low, but he wanted desperately to go home. I called his hematologist—I think it was a Sunday—and pleaded for him, saying that this guy just wants to go home. But the doctor said, "With his platelet count so low, you know what could happen to him." I said, "Yes, I know, and the patient knows, too." Finally, I convinced him to let the patient go.
>
> So he went home. He sat in the van in his driveway, and his dog came and saw him. It was the first time he had seen his dog in weeks, so he had his visit with his dog. Then they went to Taco Time, where he ate all this disgustingly fat, spicy food and threw it right up because his system couldn't handle it. He died shortly after that, but he really needed to do that—to say goodbye to his dog and his house.

Making a career decision is not only hard and emotionally taxing; it is important and exciting. For me nursing has turned out to be an exceptional choice, even though, when I made it, I felt like I was about to jump into an icy alpine lake. Standing at the edge ready to jump in, I knew I wanted to, I knew I was going to, but there was that moment of doubt, that millisecond before the jump when I thought, "You're crazy to do this!" Once I was in, though, it felt great, and my doubt was gone. Don't worry too much about your doubts; they are an inevitable part of life, and they keep you on your toes. If you do your homework, you can make an informed decision about your career based on the data you've gathered and analyzed, remembering, of course, that your emotional reactions are part of that data. Don't act on emotions alone, but don't ignore them, either.

GOING BACK FOR SECONDS: SECOND-CAREER RN

Of approximately 37% of RNs who worked in another health care area before coming to nursing, over half already had college degrees (NLN, 2006). One big advantage of second-career RNs is the experiences they bring into their nursing careers. Adults returning to school after working in another occupation are often more enthusiastic and responsible students. They make great nurses because they have experiences in their own lives that help them understand other people. They also have experiences in a workplace that help them to understand what it takes to be part of a team, to implement needed changes, and to handle conflict.

If you are worried about returning to school after an absence—fear not! Many have done so and succeeded beautifully. Nursing instructors I spoke with told me they often prefer older, returning students. One professor said, "They are more mature and know what they want. They take responsibility for their learning, which is a breath of fresh air." Another said, "They bring so much to the other students and to the patients. Their experiences make them richer people. They have understanding and tolerance. They make great nurses."

Not many people stay in the same job for their entire career anymore. In fact, in this day and age, it's not at all unusual to change jobs and even careers several times over a lifetime. The goal of receiving a gold watch, once the ideal of a lifetime of service, is dead.

Cara is a nurse practitioner. When she first became an RN she worked for several years and then decided to try being a lawyer. She went to law school and practiced as a lawyer for several years. Finally, she returned to school again to earn a master's degree as nurse practitioner. Why? She didn't like being a lawyer and missed nursing.

Gary was a chemistry teacher. Now he is a cardiac nurse. Why? He wanted more job security and was interested in science and health care. He also wanted to travel, so he and his wife, Lynnette, who is also a nurse, moved to Norway with their two children and worked in a hospital intensive care unit (ICU) for 2 years. Lynnette had a very hard time until she learned Norwegian; she loves to talk with people, and she was frustrated by using sign language. But eventually they both learned the language and loved Norway; it was a great experience for their children. (I'll talk more about traveling nurses later on in this chapter.)

Keith was a cardiovascular technician who became a nurse. Why? He wanted more challenge, more education, and more opportunity to use science.

So, if you have already gone to college, if you are working in another area, or if you want a new career, nursing may be for you. Do not discount nursing because you think you are too old for a change. One way I look at it is that at age 43 I still have at least 25 years left to work, so I'd better be doing something that I enjoy and that has a potential for personal and professional growth.

A note on returning to school: don't be afraid. There are people at the colleges whose job it is to help and support you. In fact, there's even a name for you—the "nontraditional student." These are students who have started college and left, who are older than 18 or 19, who have previous degrees, who have jobs and families, or who have various challenges such as language differences or disabilities. For instance, many Native American college students are older (considered non-traditional) students. Several Native American nurses I know became nurses in their 30's. School was a challenge because of families and moving to attend school, but they succeeded.

Nancy went to nursing school when she was 38 years old. She had two children, one a junior and the other a senior in high school. She had worked as a dental technician, as manager of the dental office, as a receptionist in a doctor's office, and finally as a medical technician in the same office. She loved working as a medical technician, and everyone kept telling her, "You need to return to school." So she did. She worked as an RN in a small hospital and as the nursing advisor at Washington State University.

I asked her why she chose nursing. She answered, "I had lived on and off in the halls of a hospital as a child. My mother had multiple sclerosis, and I helped her. I was used to the environment, and I loved the work."

It is common for people to be drawn to nursing as a result of their personal experiences with illness. Often this is good because these experiences have given you a clearer idea of what your values are or have helped you become empathetic toward others' needs. But sometimes this is not good because your experiences motivate you to go into nursing for reasons that are not really connected to being a nurse.

For example, when Robin was 25 years old and working as a teaching assistant in a preschool, she decided she wanted a change. She thought she wanted to be a nurse because she had an aunt whom she respected and admired who was a nurse. Robin thought nursing would be a good career. When she talked to the nursing adviser at her school, she said, "I like the idea of helping people. I want to do what nurses do, like giving medications, holding babies, things like that."

Robin, through no fault of her own, was basing her decision on unreal expectations, on her admiration of her aunt, and on stereotypes of nursing work. The truth is that nurses do much more than hold babies. Luckily, Robin spent a few months that summer observing a nurse in a hospital obstetrics unit. This gave her a chance to see what an obstetrics nurse really does: making complex physical, social, and cultural assessments; monitoring and following up on potential complications; coordinating all aspects of the care of a patient and her family; communicating with all other members of the health care team; and giving spiritual or grief guidance when needed. Robin changed her view of the work but still decided to major in nursing. She said, "It was different than I thought. It turned out the work was more complicated and difficult. It also turned out I liked it even more—for just those reasons."

Sydney had a degree in business from a private university where she had also played on the basketball team. After graduating, she realized she wanted to find interesting work but was unsure about what to do. She knew that there were many career opportunities in health care, so she began researching her options. She eventually chose nursing with a plan to go into a health care business. Another student, Kyle, was earning a bachelor's degree in business when he realized he was also interested in health care. He is now in nursing school getting a dual major in business and nursing. His plan is to work as an RN and then go to graduate school to become a nurse anesthetist and open his own business.

DO YOU HAVE ENOUGH GUTS TO BE A GOOD NURSE?

This is a tough question that nurses answer in a variety of ways. The Oncology Nursing Society surveyed thousands of their members as part of an effort to improve the public image of oncology nursing. The nurses were asked to choose three words that most accurately described oncology nurses. The following is a list of the five most common words:

1. Caring
2. Compassionate
3. Knowledgeable
4. Dedicated
5. Professional

My list, not in order of priority, includes these and elaborates on what I have read, observed, and gleaned from talking to nurses in a variety of fields and their patients:

THE BASICS

1. Intelligent and analytical
2. Assertive
3. Caring

4. Politically aware
5. Visionary
6. Interested in science and health
7. Seeks out and appreciates diversity
8. Creative
9. Lifelong learner
10. Culturally competent

Why these? Because nurses need to be the following:

- Leaders
- Decision makers
- Innovators—locally and globally
- Advocates for *all* kinds of people
- Teachers
- Responsible
- Caring and kind
- "People" people

In the past, the concept of the ideal nurse might have been someone who is well groomed, has his or her nursing license up to date, tests negative for tuberculosis, has no back problems, will work any shift any time, doesn't care what unit he or she is assigned to, doesn't care how much he or she is paid, is quiet, and does the work of two to three people.

A more up-to-date and realistic definition is that a nurse is a smart person who can think for herself or himself, who wants to promote the health of all people (not just certain people such as nonalcoholics, nonsmokers, or certain ethnic groups), who initiates and leads the way to needed changes, who works hard, and who cares for patients and for self (no martyrs allowed).

I asked nursing professors from Washington State University and from Gonzaga University what they wanted to see in nurses. Most named the ability to take on leadership roles as their number one most desired quality. In other words, it is absolutely vital that you consider nursing as a profession that needs assertive, thinking, committed people. Nurses who just want a pleasant or totally task-oriented job are not needed. Why? Because for one thing, with changes in health care, RNs need to be on top of the political issues that affect patients. RNs must be leaders in making sure not only that patient care is safe but that it gets the results or outcomes they want.

The National League for Nursing suggests you ask yourself the following questions to see if you have what it takes to be a nurse:

- Are you an independent, creative person?
- Can you think problems through logically?
- Do you find satisfaction in helping other people?
- Do you like math and science? Have you gotten good grades in basic math and science courses?
- Can you express yourself effectively in speech and in writing?
- Are you intrigued by machines and do you have an interest in how they work?
- Do you work well with your hands?
- Do you work well in emergency situations? Do you have common sense?
- Do you meet new people easily? Do your friends say you're a warm, friendly person? Do you prefer working around others rather than alone?

My ideal nurse is also politically active and belongs to the American Nurses Association. He or she is well read; interested in a wide variety of subjects such as music, movies, and art; living a healthy lifestyle by eating a healthy diet, exercising, and connecting to his or her culture. In short, this nurse would practice the lifestyle that she or he preached.

Reading all this, you might be thinking, "This is impossible. I might as well give up now. I could never be this ideal person." You know what? You might be that person right now. Or, if you are like me, you have these goals and values in your life and you work toward attaining them as you go. The key is this: if you have a strong interest in having these qualities, you are already on your way to being a nurse.

In summary, realize that, unless you have talked with and watched nurses on the job, you don't know what they do, because so much of nursing takes place behind the scenes (the decisions, the thinking, even the caring, are often unseen by the casual observer). So, before you decide on nursing as a career, you must find out what a nurse does by watching one at work. Then check the lists above to see if you qualify. Finally, talk to a nursing adviser at the school you wish to attend for more details.

THE DAILY GRIND: WHERE DO NURSES WORK AND WHAT DO THEY DO?

According to the Health Resources and Services Administration's 2006 *National Sample Survey of Registered Nurses*, more than half (56.2%) of all working RNs work in hospitals. The others work in public and community health (15%), ambulatory care settings such as clinics (11.5%), nursing homes and extended care facilities (6.3%), in nursing education (2.6%) or in other settings such as insurance companies, jails, health associations, or state government (8.5%).

Another 14.4% of RNs work in community or public health settings. These include health departments, visiting nurse services, home health agencies, and other nonhospital areas such substance abuse facilities.

Almost 11.5% of RNs work in ambulatory care: doctors' offices, nursing clinics, health maintenance organizations, and mixed professional practices.

Over 6% of RNs work in nursing homes or long-term care facilities. Of the rest, 2.6% work in nursing education, 2.7% in student health, 1% in occupational health, and 3% in other areas such as state boards of nursing, health planning agencies, and correctional facilities.

To give you an idea of what nurses are doing at their various work sites, RNs I interviewed shared stories that they believed represented important, or significant, moments in their careers. Not always pleasant, their stories give you insight into the thoughts, feelings, and values that are important to these nurses while they are on the job.

Crying into the Dish Towel

Sharon, a nurse practitioner, mountain-climbs, ice-skates, and is filled to the brim with fun, energy, and a wide range of interests. She has been a nurse for 21 years. While she was still in graduate school, she responded to the question, "What was a very memorable or important event in your nursing career?" with the following story:

> Shortly after graduation, I was about 25. I killed time working in a nursing home for 9 months, and then I moved back home to my rural area. My dream had always been to work in obstetrics.
>
> I worked at a 35-bed rural hospital with one labor room with two beds and an old-fashioned delivery room. We didn't have a birthing room. I got a call one night. "Sharon, we have a patient here for you, but she's not in labor." So I went in to work.
>
> The patient was a young Caucasian prime (first pregnancy) who had come in thinking she was in labor. This is fairly typical for primes. Another nurse, Terry, had

already done Leopold's maneuvers and couldn't identify the presenting part of the baby. Terry called the intern (believe me, Terry with all her vast experience would know more than the intern). But the intern couldn't figure it out either.

So they took the woman to x-ray because we didn't have ultrasound then, and there was no head. They took another x-ray. There was no head. They had a completely unexpected anencephalic baby at term in a so-called low-risk pregnancy. The reason I was called in was to give emotional support and care.

The physician was a young family practice doctor. He was devastated that he had missed this problem. And the family was devastated. I mean everyone was devastated. I still remember walking into this maelstrom of people, and the woman's father, the baby's grandfather, was intoxicated. He was being verbally abusive to the physician. I'll never forget, he was saying, "You should have known, you should have known." And I walked into this, literally to sit by the bed and help, because one of the strengths of this rural hospital was that, although we didn't have the birthing rooms or the plush carpeting, we had good one-to-one patient labor support.

I was a very new, young nurse and I was dealing with all the psychosocial needs of this family that's just been absolutely devastated. And at one point the physician offered to take me off the case because he said that we could have one of the nurses with more experience do it. I said, "No, it's okay." So, to make a long story short, inducing labor took 3 days, and we were working 12-hour shifts. I remember that I would be with her all day, sitting at the bedside running the Pitocin to promote labor, and talking, giving back rubs, just everything. And then I'd go home, and I would just sob. I still remember doing my dishes and crying into the towel. I would go back the next day because consistency of care was really important. This family and I had a good rapport. I worked to make the best out of a bad situation.

On the third day she was far enough for the physician to rupture the membranes. I never saw so much amniotic fluid in my life—gallons of it. It was just pouring over the edge of the bed, saturating the floor—you know, just pouring. And now this woman's skin over her abdomen that had been so tight and shiny was shrunken way down to nothing, like an elephant's skin.

She delivered. We were hoping that the baby would be born dead, and it was. It died right then; it never breathed. I know because I read the autopsy report later. The woman told us she didn't want to see the baby, but the husband did. We cleaned everything up; it was very traumatic for all of us. We said, "Do you still want to see the baby? It's okay if you want to. Are you ready for this?" We uncovered the baby from the feet up—you know, didn't completely expose the baby. And that father just about passed out. I mean he absolutely went white and started to get real wobbly, and I don't blame him,'cause it was beyond his worst nightmares.

I asked Sharon what she thought it took to do this kind of nursing care.

I think there's almost a conscious decision about what kind of person you are going to be, what kind of nurse you are going to be. Why did I go in on this case? There are a lot of cases like this I could tell you about. It's hard for me to remember them all. You forget about them. You take it for granted. I think we do take for granted what we do.

There was this one case where a baby died, and I had to do the postmortem care, and I am not one who likes to do that. But I remember doing that with love, like I would for my own baby, because this family was so devastated. I made the baby look as good as possible for them, because of course they couldn't do it.

But we would have fun, too. We would just laugh our guts out. We really, really had a lot of fun. I mean, we worked really hard, you know, and sometimes bizarre things would just happen.

Sharon's story is not meant to turn you away from nursing. As I said in Chapter 1, you don't have to like blood to be a nurse. Not all nurses work in such difficult circumstances, but in your training and your first years of nursing, you are likely to be working in many situations that involve pain as well as joy, life as well as death.

Trauma is Nothing Compared to This

Barb looked at me, smiled, and shook her head when I asked her to tell me a story that was typical for an ED nurse. I had asked her about working in a trauma situation such as a motor vehicle accident. She said with a great deal of authority and experience:

> You see, those aren't the situations where I think I'm most valuable. I consider that kind of stuff monkey work. Yes, it's a wonderful thing to go in there and be master in that trauma room. I shine, you know; I do it very well and very rapidly, and then I send them off to surgery. But my real nursing skill is being in a room with a woman who has been raped and knowing how to position myself in the room—where and how to sit—and to learn and understand from interview after interview that it takes 20 to 60 minutes to make her feel comfortable enough to be able to turn and make eye contact with me and eventually to talk to me about what happened. These are the skills that I consider most valuable. They're lifesaving skills. I make a tremendous difference in her life—I mean that she can either heal from this or be crippled and wounded and never heal from it for the rest of her life. People's lives are changed by the things that I do for them. And that makes me feel good.

Following in My Mother's Footsteps is Not Easy

Becky is a Nez Perce tribal member and a nurse. I interviewed her in 2002 to learn more about the experiences of Native American nurses from one of the Plateau Tribes. A tribe is considered a Plateau Tribe if it is within the Columbia Plateau, an area that includes eastern Washington state, northern Oregon, and Idaho. The following story was from an interview during which I asked Becky what she did after she first graduated from nursing school.

> As a new nurse I started working at the Nimiipuu Health Center for my tribe. I was proud of my role as a nurse in the community. I was like my mother who had been a nurse here providing an essential and unique service. A story about my mother shows what I mean.
>
> In the ER a big Indian guy was getting obnoxious, and the nurses called her and said, 'Lucy, can you come handle this?' She walked in and asked him in Nez Perce what he was doing. He looked at her and said, 'Oh, hi auntie.' She settled him down; he could relate to her. Then she tied his braid to the gurney so he couldn't move. And now they expect me to fill her shoes.
>
> Another role my mother played was as a 24-hour-a-day consultant. When mom worked nights, people would come over in the morning and wake her up. When I came home from nursing school and moved in with her, I'd tell them she was sleeping. I'd ask if I could help them. I didn't tell them I was a nurse because I didn't want to take on the burden my mother had. But when I started in the clinic and got my own housing unit, they found me and started coming. They'd say, "Can you look at my aunt?" They even brought children. I told them the ED was down the road that would be the more appropriate place to take them. People continued to drop by or call at all hours until I got an unlisted telephone number and once again moved. Despite these changes, people still found me.
>
> People thought they could come to me because of the closeness of the community. Everyone knew one another, and everyone had expectations because I was a nurse. Everybody is related in some way or another. These are the people I grew up with, and they now know I am a nurse. That is a very important position on the reservation.

Is My Baby Going to Die?

Molly, an obstetrics nurse, told me about using both her technical critical care skills and her caring skills. She finds satisfaction in caring for patients with physical and emotional needs such as the young woman and her unborn baby in this story.

A 23-year-old female presented to us at 32 weeks of a first pregnancy with complaints of headaches, blurred vision, and pitting edema. She had a nurturing and caring husband. She had gone into her doctor's office that day without any previous symptoms in her pregnancy, only to discover that she had pregnancy-induced hypertension (PIH). She was flown up to us, to an unfamiliar city without her relatives, without a support system, except her husband. We took care of her for 2 days before we decided to C-section her because her hypertension was so severe that it was starting to affect her liver and kidneys.

The environment in intensive care was not what she expected. People have their expectations on how they want their labor and delivery to occur, and sometimes these expectations are basically blown out the window. Plus she was a first-time mom, and she was wondering, "What's going to happen to my baby? Is my baby going to die?" The husband asked, "Is my wife going to die?" Hypertension causes a decreased placental flow and smaller babies. So there were a lot of variables to deal with.

She needed a lot of nurturing, caring, crisis intervention, and teaching. I told her, "We're going to take 1 hour at a time and see how things go." We wanted to see if she would display seizures or signs and symptoms of nervous system involvement such as changes in her reflexes. She grew worse, and it suddenly became a life-and-death situation for mom and baby. But we tried to stay positive and remain guardedly optimistic. We eventually stabilized her so that the C-section could be done ...everyone was fine. The baby weighed 1 pound, 6 ounces.

I enjoyed the challenge of this situation because I could be a nurturing, caring person and still use my critical care skills. I was able to impress on these people, in a gentle way, the dynamics of hypertension in a life-and-death situation. And I think they understood and were grateful.

God's in Charge

Nurses often deal with sticky moral and ethical issues that have no right or wrong answers. When a family is forced to make a life-or-death decision about their son, Tiena Lynes shows the importance nursing care plays in helping them come to grips with and resolve deeply emotional problems.

In southern California, a patient whom I'd been seeing for about 6 months had a physician who had managed his care for the past 9 years. The physician was throwing up his hands in frustration and saying that he did not want to continue with this patient anymore. His frustration was with the family, whose expectations were different from the doctor's.

The patient was this family's 31-year-old son, who had been comatose, in a vegetative state, since a gunshot wound 9 years ago. The family always wanted anything and everything done for him, but the physician did not agree with this plan of care. So I was trying to help the family find another physician. I found one, the only doctor in the entire area who would take him, but only if the family would sign a No Code, which meant that no CPR would be performed on him. But to the family that meant that they didn't love their son and that that they weren't caring for him.

I understood and respected their beliefs, but I realized that we had a cultural difference. English was not their first language. We had a person on staff who spoke Spanish, so I asked her if she would come with me on a visit and talk with the family.

My goal was to get them to sign the No Code agreement. We had a conference and talked about how signing this No Code did not mean that we would stop caring for their son. We would continue to do all that we could, but it would stop short of CPR. I managed to incorporate their belief system into the whole thing, and that was the clincher. In their belief system God was in control of their son; and if God chose to take him, then who were we to step in the way? When they understood that, even though most of the conversation was in Spanish, I could see the light come on. The mother was sitting there; she loved her dear son; she was the primary caregiver; and you could see that she understood. That felt good, very good.

Working with people in crisis situations is full of rewards and challenges. Problem solving, technical and caring skills, good communication, and careful observation are commonly used in nursing. Whether you work in a hospital or in home care, in a nursing home or in a rural clinic, these stories describe examples of the type of work you will be doing.

OPTIONS IN NURSING

In their work, nurses do just about everything you can think of. They are lawyers, businesspeople, managers, teachers, scientists, politicians, executives, business owners, inventors, exercise specialists, counselors, writers, and professional speakers.

But the very heart of nursing is patient care. It is the hands-on work of nursing in which nurse and patient interact. Even though nurses do many different things, such as teaching in nursing schools or directing a health care agency, the goals are always the same: to improve patient care and to promote health and well-being.

When you enter nursing school, you will learn all the basics of patient care. A lot of these basics include starting intravenous lines, reading heart monitors, taking blood pressures, doing physical assessments, managing medications, coordinating patient services, and patient teaching. When you get out of nursing school, you'll practice the basics. Later you may decide to get more education, work in other areas, or stay right where you are.

The following examples are not intended to show you everything nurses do, but how wide the variety is.

Flight Nurse

Peggy was a flight nurse. She worked in an intensive care unit for 4 years after graduating with her nursing degree. Then she took a job as a flight nurse. She tells this story to give an example of what can, but usually does not happen, on her job:

We received an urgent call to rescue a hiker who had fallen off a high cliff while hiking and climbing without safety ropes in the Rocky Mountains. One of the women had grabbed hold of a big rock, about the size of a medium-sized TV, but the rock pulled out of the side of the mountain. She fell backwards about 30 feet with this big rock until she hit a narrow ledge and the rock landed in her lap. One of the other climbers instantly ran to call for help. He had to run over 7 miles to find a phone that would reach an emergency service number.

Luckily, when we got the call, we had a helicopter that had just returned from refueling, so we were able to lift off immediately. When we got there, we saw one of the hikers signaling us with a piece of mirror. We flew around and saw a group of people huddled on a ledge. They waved at us, but there was no place to land. It was a sheer cliff. We had to do a one-skid landing in which one of the helicopter's skids balances on the ground while the other one is still in the air. We didn't want to take a lot of equipment with us because we had to hike down loose steep rock with no trail. So, as we landed, we threw out the C-collar, which was blown over the side of the mountain by a gust of wind, along with the airway pack and some IV gear, and climbed out after it. Then the pilot flew the helicopter about a quarter of a mile down to a meadow to wait for us.

We had to climb down to reach her. She was young and very pale, and her eyes were closed. I thought, "She's dead." So I asked somebody, "What's her name?" One of the guys crouching next to her said, "Amy." I carefully put my hand on her shoulder and shook her a little bit. I said, "Amy," expecting no response at all. Suddenly her eyes opened wide. I was so startled.

By luck, the C-collar had been blown down to the ledge, right by her side. We put it on her neck, and I started one IV—the rest of the IV stuff was still up on the top of the hill. I continued my assessment as we were preparing to move her. The only signs that I could find were a tight abdomen and a crunchy pelvis. I knew there was a pelvic abdominal injury and that she had bled a lot. I couldn't feel a pulse, and I couldn't get a blood pressure, but she had responded to her name. So that was one good sign.

I knew she was in excruciating pain. We carefully carried her hand over hand up this steep, loose slope. At the top I started another IV. She had great veins because she was an athlete; so, even though her blood pressure was so low, it was easy to start the IV.

We signaled the pilot down in the meadow to come get us. We flew back to the hospital. If she hadn't been in such good physical condition before the accident, she would have died; and if her friend hadn't been in great enough shape to run down the mountain so quickly—well, she was lucky all the way around.

Home Health Care/Community Health Nursing

Perhaps not as dramatic, but certainly equally important, is the work nurses such as Tiena and Sheila do for the Visiting Nurses Association. Sheila is the executive director, has a master's degree in nursing as an adult nurse practitioner, and is very respected in the community.

Tiena is a staff nurse with multiple roles. She teaches other nurses about the work of home care, and she sees patients in their homes. She has been a nurse for 19 years, and she loves her work because of the independence it gives her, such as making her own decisions about patient care.

One problem these nurses face is changes in insurance coverage. Community health nursing is vital, but, in an attempt to cut overall health care costs, this area is being hard hit. The problem is caused by the fact that patients need more extensive home care because they are sicker when they leave the hospitals. The solution is excellent RNs, physical therapists, respiratory therapists, and home health aides. Unfortunately, getting sufficient funding from Medicare and other insurance companies to cover the cost of home care can be a problem. But this is also an area where nurses have been lobbying heavily for change.

Researcher

Ora L. Strickland is an African-American nurse. I highlight this fact because African-Americans are a minority in nursing, and yet, historically and presently, they've made major contributions to nursing. Dr. Strickland received her bachelor's degree in nursing from North Carolina Agricultural and Technical State University, a master's degree from Boston University, and a doctorate in child development and family relations from the University of North Carolina.

Through the use of her research findings, which influence changes in health policies on a national and international level, she has the power to improve the health of women and children. She has researched breast cancer in African-American women and created cultural and age-sensitive guidelines for the National Institutes of Health in the largest long-term study of women ever conducted. She has studied how men respond to their wives' pregnancies, and she has done groundbreaking work on the physiology of PMS. She is an example of a powerful nurse and a powerful human being who is using her intelligence and caring to solve problems for her profession and for society.

There are other nurses who do valuable research. Many of these teach in universities or work for the government, for nonprofit foundations, for clinics, for physicians, and for themselves. International nursing organizations such as Sigma Theta Tau support nursing scholarship and research.

Hospital Obstetrics Nurse

Molly has worked in many areas of the hospital, including the surgical unit, intensive care unit, and now in obstetrics. She loves this work the best. She says, "I get to use all my skills here. Everything I learned in the other areas is combined here." She works with mothers, babies, and family members during tragedies and celebrations. She is widely appreciated and loved by her patients for her work with them during difficult times. One new mother who also happens to be a nurse, told me, "Molly is the best nurse I know. She is caring and smart."

Family Nurse Practitioner

Maria decided to be a nurse just after she earned her bachelor's degree in history when she realized that she was going to have a tough time finding a job. When she visited a friend whose mother was a rural home care nurse, she realized that this was the type of work she wanted to do. She had always wanted a job with independence and she liked the idea of working with people. So she returned to school for 2 more years to earn a second bachelor's degree, this time in nursing. That was 16 years ago. Since that time she's worked in emergency and cardiac care. Now, after another 2 years of school, she has a master's degree in nursing, with certification as a family nurse practitioner.

She works with a family practice physician and two other nurse practitioners. She loves her work because she has authority and independence. She uses her science background, works with people, and has a sense that she is doing work that makes a difference in other people's lives.

Operating Room Anesthesia

Janelle has been a nurse for "a very long time." She earned a diploma degree in nursing from a hospital nursing program and later a bachelor's and a master's degree from a university. She is a certified registered nurse anesthetist, or a CRNA. She provides anesthesia to patients receiving open-heart surgery, and she goes to the labor and delivery unit to give spinal anesthesia to women having babies. Janelle is highly respected by the hospital staff and especially by the women having babies.

Oncology Nurse

Stefanie has been a nurse for 10 years. She is 28 years old, has a 3-year-old daughter, and is planning a wedding. She graduated from a 2-year associate's degree program in nursing and went to work in the intensive care unit of a small hospital. Now she's back at a university to earn a bachelor's degree in nursing. Stefanie survived her own bout with cancer, an advanced-stage lymphoma, and now her goal is to work with other cancer patients.

She works part-time for a cancer clinic and plans to go full-time after she completes her degree. Stefanie is energetic, cheerful, intelligent, and creative. She is brimming with good ideas, both for her patients and for the profession of nursing. She takes time to write to her state representatives and senators about health care and nursing issues, and recently she organized a successful "Cancer Survivors Day" in her community. She has a great career ahead of her.

Case Manager

Kate has worked in home health and in intensive care. She also worked for a large health maintenance organization as a case, or care resource, manager. In this capacity she managed a large group of patients after first seeing them in the hospital to assess their needs and then again after they were discharged. She has saved her organization, and health care as a whole, money. Nurses in case management are helping in major ways to decrease health care costs by following patients from illness to health and making sure that all goes smoothly along the way. There is impressive research showing that nurse case managers lower the number of patients that have to be readmitted to the hospital for infections or other complications.

As important as saving money is, equally important is the intangible aspect—the human side of things. Who wants to go back to the hospital? Isn't once enough? So Kate in her nursing practice is a money saver, a health promoter, and a humanitarian.

This list could go on and on. There are many kinds of nursing I left out. Can you think of any? What interests you? Do any of the above sound appealing?

Well, hang on, because you're about to get a look at the terrain ahead and a first-hand view of the rewards and problems of being a nurse. After that, in the next chapter, we will get a bit more practical and take a good look at schools, licensing, and finding jobs.

COOL, CLEAR, AND TOXIN FREE: NURSING'S REWARDS

Nursing is by no means a boring profession, and there is work to do at every level. One level involves keeping the profession healthy by being active in professional associations such as the American Nurses Association. This work promotes nursing, as well as all kinds of health care issues, from child health to gun control to AIDS. Another level is direct patient care such as that done by a critical care nurse in a hospital who might care for someone with gunshot wounds, life-threatening tuberculosis, sudden cardiac death, or an HIV-positive drug addict. Nurses do it all. I think nurses have it all as well. In other words, the rewards of being a nurse are many and diverse, including helping others live more healthful lives.

The following sections outline a few examples of the rewards of nursing.

Job Security

The National League for Nursing (NLN) reports most nursing school graduates have a job lined up at the time of graduation, the rest in less than 4 months. You may get your first job in a nursing home or other nonhospital setting. If you are really interested in working in a hospital, you are likely to get the job you want, with a few exceptions. Some positions are not open to new nursing graduates. For instance, Tim wants to work in pediatric oncology, but he will have to work in another area— perhaps adult oncology—for a few years. Another graduating student wants to work in the pediatric intensive care unit but will work in a regular pediatrics unit first.

Travel

Nurses can and do work anywhere in the world. You can move to places like Kenya, Paris, Australia or Denver, Colorado. There are many traveling nurse organizations such as Cross Country TravCorps that employ nurses and send them around the world (see websites in Appendix A). If you work in a foreign country, you won't need to know another language; but, unless you work in an American or military hospital, it can help. Gary and Lynnette, who worked in a Norwegian intensive care unit, were hired and worked for 2 years there with no previous knowledge of the language.

Money

As I said, the average salary for a nurse in 2004 (the most recent federal statistics) is close to $58,000 a year (HRSA 2006). It has risen even higher since then.

Flexibility

Need to work at night so you can go to school during the day or be home for your kids before and after school? Need to work evenings because you hate to get up early? Need to work short days, for example 7 AM to noon? Nursing offers amazing flexibility in the hours you can work. Nurses are needed in many places 24 hours a day, 7 days a week, holidays included; thus creative staffing is encouraged to increase job satisfaction.

Many nurses work 12-hour shifts. Those are long, tiring hours, but how does 7 to 9 days off sound? Or how does it sound to work three 12-hour shifts on Friday, Saturday, and Sunday and have the rest of the week off?

Personal Reward

The nurses I interviewed thought, without a doubt, that nursing brought a great deal of value into their lives. They found nursing satisfying and rewarding, which is pretty amazing if you think about how many people you know who don't feel this way about their work. And it's a good thing, too, for both the nurse and the patient. A recent nursing study correlated job satisfaction with patient outcomes: the more satisfied nurses were on the job, the fewer the complications, such as infections, that occurred among the patients.

If you think about how long you will be working, job satisfaction and personal rewards begin to increase in importance. The age you become eligible to receive Medicare is expected to be raised to 67 years old. Try this: 67 – your age = _____, the number of years left to work. If you're 18 years old that's 49 years. 25 years old? That's 42 more years—my whole lifetime. Wow!

Prestige and Respect

Prestige depends on your perspective. It's like looking at a view. If you love skiing, the view of a huge mountain slope covered in luscious, new powdery snow is a dream come true that can make your mouth water. On the other hand, if you hate winter, can't tolerate cold, and hate skiing, the view makes you nauseous. Life is just like this. The way you see the view depends on what you value.

Some of the things I value are service to others, good health, science and research, and persistent inquiry. These infuse my view of nursing with fantastic reward and prestige. Take a moment to think about what you value, locally and globally, and remember the praises the World Health Organization has heaped on nursing in its "indispensable" role in the health of nations.

IS THERE A PROBLEM?

Many of nursing's problems stem from its history. Taking care of people when they are sick has typically been thought of as women's work, and women's work (which has usually included teaching, secretarial work, and homemaking) has generally been underpaid and undervalued. For instance, nurses often take a back seat to doctors. It is not uncommon for people to think of nurses as assistants to doctors, an idea that is not true. The good news is that nurses, recognizing these inequities, have grown tired of bemoaning low pay and low status, or worse, just putting up with it, and are working hard to gain more control over the direction in which the profession and, for that matter, health care as a whole are going.

Nurses are doing this by taking political action to effect changes in laws governing the payment of nurses for their services and by mounting public awareness campaigns to make nursing more visible, better understood, and hence more highly valued. This has been done through highlighting achievements in research, publication, public speaking, and the media.

To increase the understanding of what nurses do and how nurses are necessary for safe, quality care, nursing researchers are showing what nurses have feared—patients suffer when the number of RNs decreases. Hospitals with a ratio of fewer RNs to patients tend to have more patient complications, which, of course, costs more money and negates any savings intended by cutting RNs in the first place. Hospitals that assign a RN too many patients find safety and quality at risk. There is also growing evidence that an RN's education level affects care. Linda Aiken has gained well deserved recognition for her study of surgical patients cared for by RNs with associate degrees (community college) and bachelor's degrees (university). She and her research team discovered that the patients cared for by bachelor-prepared nurses had fewer complications.

In the political arena, battles are being fought and won by the American Nurses Association and other nursing groups. Medicare legislation provides that nurse practitioners may receive direct reimbursement for services they are legally authorized to perform under state nurse practice acts. Workplace violence is an issue faced by all health care workers. Nurses are lobbying for better federal standards to protect nurses, doing research, and working with other groups on education.

Mandatory overtime legislation has been passed in some states to prevent forcing nurses to work when they are overly tired. This is a patient safety issue. Nurses (or anyone for that matter) are unable to think as clearly as needed when they have worked too long. Currently some states allow forcing nurses to work overtime. If a nurse refuses, he or she can actually be fired or lose his or her license. In a real emergency, overtime is needed, but in many cases overtime is used as a way to meet routine staffing shortages.

The American Nurses Association's Department of Government Affairs notes the following in its initiatives for the 109th Congress:*

A recent ANA survey of nearly 5000 nurses across the nation revealed that more than 67% are working unplanned overtime every month. Research shows that sleep loss influences several aspects of performance, leading to slowed reaction time, delayed responses, failure to respond when appropriate, false responses, slowed thinking, diminished memory and others. In fact, 1997 research conducted at the University of Australia showed that work performance is more likely to be impaired by moderate fatigue than by alcohol consumption. It is well understood that significant safety risks are posed by fatigued workers.

*American Nurses Association (ANA). (2006). *Nursing's legislative and regulatory initiatives for the 109th Congress.* Silver Spring, Md: ANA.

Another important nursing political and social issue is the number of people in the United States without health insurance. Susan Trossman wrote the following in the *American Journal of Nursing:*[†]

Last year, paramedics brought a young, uninsured African-American man to a Chicago ED in full respiratory arrest. Despite their efforts, nurses and physicians could not revive him.

His death was a tragedy, compounded by the fact that it could have been prevented, according to Illinois Nurses Association (INA) president Mary Maryland, PhD, RN, APRN, BC. Nurses found prescriptions in his pocket for asthma medications he had received during an earlier visit to the same ED. Without insurance, he couldn't afford to fill them.

Like other nurses, Maryland has many stories about the uninsured, who number about 1.7 million in Illinois and 41.2 million in the United States. And at a Chicago town hall meeting March 10, the first day of Cover the Uninsured Week, she shared the story of the young man who frequented the ED for his care, as well as strategies she believes will ease this growing health care crisis.

FACTS ABOUT THE UNINSURED[‡]
- Eight of 10 uninsured Americans come from working families who either have no health coverage through their employer or cannot afford insurance when it's offered.
- Nearly 20% of the uninsured are children, and those most likely to lack health care coverage are between 18 and 24 years old.
- Over one-third of uninsured adults did not fill a drug prescription or went without a test or treatment due to cost.
- Every 30 seconds an American files for bankruptcy after having a health problem.
- The U.S. spends more on health care than any other industrialized nation, but is the *only* one that does not have a unified national health care plan.

This brings us to an issue that has been with nursing a long time—workplace problems such as communication between nurses and physicians. You can ask any nurse, and you are sure to be given examples of being yelled at by doctors, having the phone hung up, being laughed at, and even being sexually harassed. Such incidents are humiliating and on a day-to-day basis can add significantly to a nurse's level of fatigue. I know from talking to nurses that these problems still exist but that sexual harassment has decreased significantly due to legislation, increased awareness education, and the potential any employer faces of being sued for allowing abuse to be inflicted on employees.

Many doctors understand the importance of a health care team in which each member has an equally important role, and they are great to work with. Studies have shown that nurses want to have collaborative relationships with doctors, but that the reverse is not always true. Nurse-doctor relations constitute one of the problems in nursing that you will learn to deal with not as a victim, but through action. You will learn how to handle conflict, how to communicate effectively, and when to seek the help of your supervisors.

[†]Trossman S. (2003). Health care for all. *American Journal of Nursing, 103*(7):77-79, 2003.
[‡]From: RESULTS: http://www.results.org/website/article.asp?id=1563

Another problem in nursing is more personal. Nursing advisers will tell students that in order to become a nurse it takes more than the simple desire to want to help people. They say this because it is not uncommon for people with past health problems, their own or their family's, to want to go into nursing as a way to give something back. If you think you might fit in this category, examine your expectations and realize that, although nursing is rewarding and satisfying, it requires much more than a desire to help. Nurses are not at work to hammer out their personal problems. In fact, you can hurt yourself, others, and the profession if this is your motivation.

On the other hand, your problems can be a source of understanding. A student who was paralyzed from the waist down wanted to be a nurse. She thought she would be good at understanding what other people with spinal cord injuries were going through. She understood that there were many mental and emotional adjustments (what nurses call psychosocial) that go along with a devastating injury. She was clear about her values, and she understood her own problems. Her experiences have helped her develop empathy—a vital component of being a great nurse.

Nurses have a tall order for the 21st century—changing the health care system—but it's one that there're up to, and you must be, too, if you decide to become a nurse. The problems are sky high, but so are the rewards. Nursing requires brainpower, but I think that's why we have these big brains—to use them! It's what makes us both human and humanitarians. Making the world a better place is an admirable choice, don't you think?

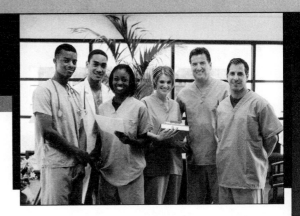

How to Get Where You Want to Go

GETTING STARTED

If you are reading this book, you might have a good idea of what your goals are and that you want to be a nurse. On the other hand, you may be trying to get an idea of what you want to do. This chapter will help you figure that out.

Step 1: Mission, Vision, and Goals

Understanding your basic values, or what you hold to be important, is the first step in deciding what you want to do. Whatever career you choose, you want it to fit your values. Then you can use your values to guide you in writing a mission and vision statement. Writing this statement reinforces your focus as you continue in your education.

You may think this is an unnecessary step because you know what you want to do. But writing your goals down will make you clarify your thoughts. This will help you in discussions with others as you progress in college and apply to nursing school. To be able to say what you want or where you want to go is a crucial step toward making it happen. Start with your values.

Step 2: Values (What Do I Think is Important?)

Write down as many things as you can that you value. Then prioritize about 10 of them. This is not an easy exercise, and your answers can change over time. It is difficult to say what is most important, but remember that your list is not written in stone. It is a way to clarify your thinking that will help you make decisions about your future.

For example, my values list (not necessarily in order of importance) reads as follows:
- Education
- Learning
- Reading
- Gardening
- Time with family
- Time with friends
- Social justice
- Equity
- Movies
- Art
- Honesty
- Integrity
- Humor

Following is the statement of core values for my college:

The Washington State University Intercollegiate College of Nursing embraces the core values of caring, altruism, social justice and maximizing human potential. In addition, the College endorses the values of Washington State University and the consortium institutions, Eastern Washington University, Gonzaga University and Whitworth College that include inquiry and knowledge, engagement and application, committed partnerships, leadership, character, stewardship, teamwork and diversity. (Retrieved April 18, 2006, from http://nursing.wsu.edu/administration/splan.asp.)

Now prioritize your values. Start with what is most important to you. This will be difficult, but give it a shot! Remember that you can change later. Some of my priorities are:
1. Social justice
2. Time with family

3. Education and learning
4. Time with friends
5. Humor

Step 3: Develop a Mission That's Possible

You can write your mission using the college of nursing's mission and my mission as examples. Or use other examples, including your own ideas. Mission statements are usually based on your values, so use yours to write your mission statement.

My mission is to advocate for vulnerable people and environments by promoting the health and well-being of all people and places. My professional mission is to promote the values of the nursing profession of advocacy and care through local and international efforts. I plan to enjoy life through art and humor and caring for myself, my family, and my friends.

Following is the mission statement for the WSU College of Nursing:

> The Washington State University Intercollegiate College of Nursing is committed to inspiring and transforming health care for generations to come. (Retrieved April 18, 2006, from http://nursing.wsu.edu/administration/splan.asp.)

Step 4: Write Your Vision to See a Long Way Ahead

Let your vision be as broad and big as you want it to be. Let it be grand or small, complicated or simple. Most of all, let it reflect who you are. If you are creative, you can turn this into an art project. Instead of just writing your vision, create it: paint; draw; sculpt it out of clay, objects, or paper. A vision is what you see happening, and it includes your mission. The following is an example of an organizational vision; yours, of course, will be personal.

> The Washington State University Intercollegiate College of Nursing pursues opportunities to expand the frontiers of nursing knowledge, science and practice. Using innovative technological approaches, integrated teaching and research, and leveraged resources to benefit all people, the College bridges barriers to health care in the global community with a focus on underserved and rural populations. (Retrieved April 18, 2006, from http://nursing.wsu.edu/administration/splan.asp.)

> *Nursing's Agenda for the Future*,* developed in 2002 by nursing leaders, gave the following as its 2010 vision:

> Nursing is *the* pivotal health care profession, highly valued for its specialized knowledge, skill and caring in improving the health status of the public and ensuring safe, effective, quality care. The profession mirrors the diverse population it serves and provides leadership to create positive changes in health policy and delivery systems. Individuals choose nursing as a career, and remain in the profession, because of the opportunities for personal and professional growth, supportive work environments and compensation commensurate with roles and responsibilities.

Step 5: Write Down Your Long-Term Goals

Long- term goals are what you want to accomplish over months or years. Short-term goals are the smaller steps that will help you reach them. Setting long-term goals

---

*The entire document *Nursing's Agenda for the Future* can be downloaded from www.nursingworld.org/naf/.

will help you make a plan. Long-term goals can be of varying lengths, from months, to a year, to a lifetime. Begin by writing two long-term goals. Following is an example of two goals that will take several years:

1. I will be admitted to the college of my choice, ready to study and succeed in learning.
2. I will graduate with a degree in nursing prepared to work in a career that will help people in my community live better lives.

Step 6: Write Down Your Short-Term Goals

Short-term goals will help you reach long-term goals. Makes sense, doesn't it? Short-term goals can be really specific and can be for just 1 day or several. A short-term goal I have for this week is to walk 4 miles three times. My short-term goal for today is to finish writing this chapter and then go for one of those walks! The following are examples of other short-term goals related to the long-term goals in Step 5. Write several short-term goals to help you reach one of your long-term goals.

1. I will get a B or higher for a grade in my science class.
2. I will finish my lab write-up today.
3. I will study for 2 hours on Monday, Tuesday, Wednesday and for 1 hour on Thursday.

Another way to use goal setting is for longer projects. For example, you have to be prepared to present a lab project you did in science to your entire class in 2 weeks.

The long-term goal will be: _____.

The short-term goals will be:

1. Two weeks from now I will _____.
2. One week from now I will _____.
3. Today by the end of the day I will _____.
4. By 3 PM today I will _____.

Notice how all the goals are connected and how they support each other. Then notice how your goals support your values and your mission. Can you see a connection with your vision? As you do these exercise, don't forget your personal health goals. As a nurse, or any other professional, you will have to be able to care for yourself in order to care for others. If you are not healthy or if you are tired or cranky, you will not be a safe or effective nurse. Do what you can to keep body and mind at their best.

ON TO COLLEGE:
WHAT TO EXPECT AND STRATEGIES TO SUCCEED

The first thing to expect when thinking about college is a certain amount of fear mixed with excitement. If you are just going off to college, it may be your first time away from home, your first time doing things on your own. If you have already been to college and are now returning after an absence, you will also be experiencing a big change. One student applying to nursing school said that the best example of her ability to adapt to change was her college experience. She deliberately chose a school far from home because she wanted to find out what it was like. She said she was scared at first but realized how much she learned about herself and how much confidence she gained.

Depending on where you go, the amount of change you experience will vary. If you are from a small community and go away to college, the experience of being around lots of people you don't know will be a big change. If you are a student from another country, from a culture that is not well represented at the college, or if you have characteristics that you think are especially unique—college can be a big change. Probably the main thing all students have in common is the change college life represents.

Strategies for Success
This section will cover strategies to help you succeed. It is an overview and not intended to tell you everything. Begin by asking the questions outlined in the following discussion.

Strategy No. 1: Who Can Help Me?
You will want to start by thinking about people who can help you in some way. Who might that be? It could be anyone who is smart, caring, or willing to encourage you. It can be more than one person and might include one or more of the following:
- A parent or other relative
- A teacher or counselor
- Someone who is in the profession you are thinking about going into, perhaps a nurse
- A person in your community who is an elder, a leader, or scholar
- A friend

Strategy No. 2: What Can College Do For Me?
Why do you want to go to college? To get a good job? To learn another language? To travel abroad? To meet new people? To get away from home? To learn how to better help the people from your home? There are many reasons to go to college. A primary reason may be the financial advantage college graduates gain in the workplace. It is true that in the United States college graduates make higher salaries than those who do not graduate, but a college degree alone doesn't guarantee a higher salary. You have to make the most of it.

You should go to college for the sake of education, not just to get a job. A good liberal arts background will help you in the workplace. Studies have shown that students who receive a 4-year college degree from a good liberal arts college do better in the workplace in terms of being flexible and adaptable to change and being able to creatively problem solve. These are highly desirable traits in the eyes of employers.

Take the opportunity of being at college to learn about many things such as different cultures, art, literature, and music. The following two exercises may help you make your decision:
1. Make a list of all the things you think you could learn and gain by attending college. If you get stuck or want more information, try the next exercise.
2. Interview a college graduate. Go to your local health clinic and talk to a nurse, a nurse practitioner, a doctor, or a pharmacist. Ask that person why he or she would recommend college to you. Write down the answers to look back on later.

Strategy No. 3: What's What?
To learn what you will be expected to do in college, begin by figuring out the basic college requirements. How many credits will you need to graduate? What courses do you need to get into nursing school? Next figure out how to calculate your grade point average (GPA).

| Converting a Letter Grade to a Number ||
Letter Grade	Number Grade
A	4.0
A–	3.7
B+	3.3
B	3.0
B–	2.7
C+	2.3
C	2.0
C–	1.7
D+	1.3
D	1.0
F	0.0

Calculate GPA

Write down the course name, the number of credits or hours, the letter grade, and the number grade. Next, multiple the number of credits by the number grade. Add those up and divide by the total number of credits or hours.

Biology I	5	B	3.0 (3.0 × 5) = 15.0
Spanish II	5	A–	3.7 (3.7 × 5) = 18.5
Social Justice	2	C	2.0 (2.0 × 2) = 4.0
Freshman Writing	3	B–	2.7 (2.7 × 3) = 8.1
TOTAL HOURS/CREDITS	15		45.6

Total numeric grade = 45.6
Divide by hours/credits:

45.6 ÷ 15 = 3.04

Looking at the chart above you can see that you would have a 3.0 GPA, or a B average.

Strategy No. 4: Who Does What on the College Campus, and What Can They Do for Me?

Start with the Administration. Many large schools have different departments with different administrative staff. A college nursing program will have a dean who oversees that college. The university also has a president, vice presidents, and others whose job it is to further the mission of teaching. The following is a list of people and places to begin to gather information about the college nursing program.

- *The Office of Student Affairs*: They can answer questions and provide support.
- *The Registrar's Office*: They handle registration and send out grades and transcripts.
- *The Financial Aid Office*: They will help you apply for financial aid and give you information about what types of aid you might qualify for.
- *The Bursar's Office or Finance, Accounting, Cashiering*: The people in this office issue bills for your tuition, room, and board.
- *Student Services*: From the school's web page, you can usually find a list of student services. These are important to you. Examples include Student Health;

Computer Center; Career Services; Multicultural Centers; and student groups such as Gay, Lesbian Bisexual, Transgendered (GLBT), Native American, Latino, African-American; Asian-American, International, Disabled, and Veteran's Affairs.

Strategy No. 5: How Can I Improve my Critical Thinking Fitness Level?

Questioning, identifying, comparing, and forming and testing a hypothesis are examples of critical thinking. In college, and throughout life, you will need to have a critical thinking fitness plan along with your physical fitness plan. Nurses need excellent critical thinking fitness. An example follows.

A patient arrives in the Emergency Department (ED) and you, the registered nurse, are the first to assess her. The patient is a teenager who says she took too many pain pills. You ask what kind of pills, and she says she doesn't remember. So what do you do now? THINK CRITICALLY.

- *Ask questions:* What is the policy in the ED for possible overdoses? Does the patient have a family member who can find out quickly what pills she took? Ask the patient why she took the pills?
- *Identify:* You must begin to identify the problems and then prioritize them. You must identify the patient's blood pressure and other physical and mental signs.
- *Compare:* How is this patient similar to or different from other patients you have seen with similar problems? Compare this situation with the clinical guidelines for working with male teens.
- *Form and test a hypothesis:* From the information you have gathered (the patient's report of symptoms and history, the family, your own assessment, your past experience, and your knowledge of evidenced-based practice) you form a possible answer, or hypothesis. You know the patient took the drug several hours ago, you know she took aspirin, you know she had a headache, you can see that her physical signs are normal, and you know you do not want to order a lot of unnecessary tests. Therefore your hypothesis is that the patient is looking for attention. You decide to test this hypothesis. What do you do next? What do you want to make sure you don't overlook?

This is just one example of the need for excellent critical thinking fitness. As a nurse you will be running mental marathons, and you will have a great deal of responsibility for the results. You begin to train by going to college and showing up for class. Getting engaged in the school work and talking to others about important issues and problems will also really help you learn critical thinking.

Strategy No. 6: How Can I Succeed at Studying, Taking Notes, Writing, and Taking Tests?

You do not automatically know how to study. Effective study skills are learned, hopefully throughout your school years, including high school. Students coming into the college of nursing where I teach have very high grade point averages. Tyson, a nursing student, said that after his first test in nursing school he realized he didn't really know how to study. He was a very bright student who had managed to get a 3.8 GPA his first 2 years of college without studying very rigorously. He soon found out that he had to learn a better way to take notes in class, study, write, and take tests. Following are some tips for each of these:

1. *Studying: You Cannot Cram*

   You will not be able to remember the amount of information you need in college or nursing school no matter how smart you are. Study everyday you have a class. If you have class on Wednesday, study Wednesday evening. If the class meets again on Friday, review for it Thursday night and study Friday after class. Basically, you study frequently for shorter time periods. "Cramming," or studying all night before a test, may work in some situations, but it is a terrible way to learn, and more important for a test, to remember.

Memory works best if fed small amounts frequently over time. Does this sound familiar? Yes, it is a good way to eat too! One good way to study after class is to recopy your notes. One good way to study before class is to skim the readings. Look for chapter headings and subheadings. Make the subheading into a question. For example, a subheading in this book is 'College: What to Expect and Strategies to Succeed.' Turn that into a question and answer it. What are three things I should expect in college? What are three strategies I can use to succeed in college? Read the book to answer those questions. This method keeps you from getting too involved in reading details when you don't have time.

2. *Note-Taking*

The key to note taking is to take notes. Sounds obvious, but students who take classes with detailed preprepared outlines or who use PowerPoint slides with copies online do not always take notes. They rely on the slides. Writing things down is another way to help it get into your memory for later use. The simple act of taking notes actually increases what you remember. Then, and this is the wonderful thing about note taking, when you recopy the notes later, your memory is even more likely to retain the information.

There are numerous note-taking systems. You may have one you use already. You can go to your student services academic center, learning specialist, or counselor to find other systems.

3. *Writing Papers*

Writing is a skill. It is learned over time and with practice just like you learn to play a musical instrument, speak a language, or paint a picture. Writing a paper and making a presentation are similar in the following ways.

a. You need to know who your audience is. For whom is the paper or presentation intended? If you are presenting to a group of elementary children about bicycle safety, your presentation will be different than if you are presenting to a group of college students. If you are writing a research paper about heart disease for your professor, it will be different than if you were writing a newsletter article on the same topic for a local senior center. Audiences vary by how much they know or want to know about your topic. They also vary by how much they want to hear about the topic. You may have to spend most of the presentation engaging them, or convincing them that they do want to hear about the topic.

b. What is the purpose of the presentation or paper? Is it to inform, to persuade, to inspire action? The type of language you use is influenced by this purpose. To inform someone, you present facts. To persuade, you create an argument backed up with facts.

c. You can find many resources for learning to write a good research or scholarly paper for college courses. But I have some tips. Remember that for most college papers you are not expressing your opinion outright. You may have an opinion, but in the paper you want it to look like you are just presenting the facts. Avoid use of qualifying words such as "terrible" or "fantastic" or other words that denote your opinion. Use lots of references to back up what you write. Research the topic so that you present the latest findings.

d. Finally, plan on writing four to five drafts. Unless the paper is simply meant to be your opinion about something (generally the easiest kind of paper to write), rewrite often. Get someone else to read the paper and make corrections. Another great idea is to read it out loud to someone or to yourself. Saying it aloud will help you catch errors very quickly.

4. *Giving Presentations*

Like writing a paper, you need to know who your audience is. Will it be your peers or a community group? Here are the basics for a presentation. You can follow this outline for any kind of presentation you need to give. The following is adapted from a great book, though old, by Leon Fletcher, *How To Speak Like a Pro* (New York, 1983, Ballantine Books). I give many presentations, and it hasn't failed me yet.

a. The introduction: about 15% of your allotted time
   Include an attention-getting opener such as a question or startling fact and a preview of what you are going to say.

b. The discussion: about 75% of the allotted time
   Make your main points here in some kind of logical order and use data to back them up.

c. The conclusion: about 10% of allotted time
   Summarize what you said and compose a memorable ending using a quote or the "take home" message.

Finally, there is always some stage fright. Many people are really afraid to speak in public and feel they would rather die. Any irrational fear such as this is called a *phobia*. If you have a phobia of speaking in public, you are not alone! But you can overcome it. You may never enjoy public speaking, but you might become more comfortable! My ideas for getting more comfortable follow.

a. Be prepared. Practice your presentation by giving it first just to yourself and then to trusted friend (or maybe even your trusted pet).

b. If you can, use PowerPoint slides or some other visual aid. This takes the attention away from you, and you can do it in a darkened room if necessary. The slides also act as cues for what to say next.

c. Talk to your teacher and tell him or her how you feel. Remember that you are not alone and your teacher will not think you are crazy—rather, he or she will help you!

d. Even the most seasoned public speakers get stage fright.

A friend from the Colville Confederated Tribes told me the hardest part of nursing school was public speaking. She said she had always been a quiet person, not used to speaking out. She told me what helped her was something her elders told her. They advised her to always speak from her heart. That worked for my friend who now speaks often in public.

5. *Taking Tests*

Here is my take-home message about taking tests. Being a good test taker does not mean you are smarter than those who are not good test takers. Also, having difficulty taking tests has nothing to do with how good a nurse you will be. Test taking is a skill that some people are good at and others not so good.

If you have trouble with tests, go to your school's learning center and ask for help. There is a great deal of tried and true information on how to become a better test taker.

Read one of the many books on how to be a better test taker. Do not use your difficulty taking tests to assume that you cannot go to college, succeed in college, or become a nurse. Anytime you have trouble with academics, get help. There are tutors, learning specialists, and counselors. Their jobs rely on people like you, and they have lots of experience helping people succeed.

Strategy No. 7: How Can I Build a Community of Support?

Everyone needs help. Are you thinking of becoming a nurse because you think you might want to help people? There are lots of people who like to help people. This means there are lots of people who would like to help you. You may already know that, but if you don't, just think about it. You need to learn to be able to ask for help. Who do you know who thinks your idea of going to college and becoming a nurse is a good one? Start with that person. Then think of someone you know who is a nurse; if you don't know one, ask around. You can go to your local clinic or your college health center.

If you are a student of color or an international student, it is great to have a role model from your community. This person can talk to about how he or she managed college, about what it was like for him or her to leave home, and what it has been like to return to the community as a nurse. Many cultures have different views on education. These can include ideas on whether women should leave home to go to college, whether men should become nurses, or about what happens when you go to a college where the majority of students are Caucasian. Talking to people who have already accomplished what you are hoping to can be a great source of support.

Find the multicultural center on your campus. Make contact with people from your community. The kind of support you can find by being with people you feel comfortable with or with people who have had similar experiences can reduce the stress of college in a significant way (there is even research to back this up). Seek support even if you think you don't need it. That may sound strange, but even if you don't think you need it now, you will need it sometime. Get possible support people lined up so that, when the time comes, you know what to do!

DIVERSITY AT COLLEGE AND WITHIN NURSING

You probably already know that diversity among people is not only about ethnicity or skin color. There is diversity in gender, physical abilities, religion, intelligence, communication, and learning styles. Diversity on a college campus makes learning a richer experience for everyone. Diversity on work teams increases group effectiveness. When you have people with different ideas and ways of doing things, the chances for group success increases.

In nursing and in health care, diversity is important because the populations we serve are diverse. Health care providers need to reflect the population. If you want to see a female or a male doctor only because you feel more comfortable and not because they will do a better job, you should be able to do so. If the person is not available in your community, your choices and comfort level are decreased. It is important for people to feel comfortable with their health care professionals in their own communities.

As noted in Chapter 1, nursing is the most ethnically diverse health care profession, but it does not reflect the ethnic diversity of the U.S. population. About 88% of nurses are non-Hispanic Caucasians. The U.S. population is only 70% non-Hispanic Caucasians (2004 National Sample Survey of Registered Nurses HRSA 2006 http://bhpr.hrsa.gov/healthworkforce/reports/rnpopulation/preliminaryfindings.htm). One reason to increase ethnic diversity in nursing is to provide culturally competent care. Culturally competent care can be provided by a nurse of any ethnicity to any patient, but if a patient wants a nurse who is of a similar ethnicity, he or she needs to have that choice.

Cultural competence means showing respect for those of different cultures. It means being able to ask sensitive questions in sensitive settings. It means knowing the critical importance of having trained interpreters available for non-English speaking patients. It also means being able to understand the patient's perspective. Think about this—what is health? Is it a perception? How do you know you are healthy? How do you know when you are sick? What do you do if you are sick? To whom do you talk? To whom do you go to for help? When do you go for help? What does being sick mean to you? If you really think about these questions, you will see that they are culturally based. You learn culture; and you learn what to consider healthy or sick, when to go for help, and to whom to go. What it means to be sick is also something that comes from your own experiences. The Office of Minority Health of the U.S. Department of Health and Human Services has published Guidelines for Cultural Competency in Health Care, available at www.omhrc.gov/.

You can understand why a nurse needs to understand these concepts about health. Knowledge about culture and health is necessary to be a good nurse and to provide the highest quality care. Nurses need to be able to understand their patients; they need to be able to communicate with their patients. Without cultural competency, nurses cannot communicate well with patients other than those from their own age, gender, or ethnic group.

5

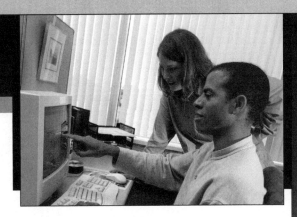

The Five Rights: Choosing the Right School

The five rights are basic safety rules for giving medications and one of the first things you will learn in nursing school. They are right patient, right drug, right dose, right time, and right route. In this chapter, we're concerned with the five levels of nursing education and how you decide which one is right for you. With a high school education you can enter three of the five levels—diploma, associate's degree, or bachelor's degree; whereas the other two (master's degree and doctoral degree) require a college degree. The following list explains the first three levels in greater depth:

- *Diploma of nursing:* In some parts of the country, hospital nursing programs at this level still exist whereby you can earn a diploma of nursing in 3 years. These programs are run by hospital boards of trustees; and most, if not all, of the training is done in their facility. Diploma schools cannot grant college credits for the classes you take; thus if you think further education is a possibility, careful consideration of other options is needed. Some diploma schools are affiliated with colleges to give you credit for at least the basic science courses, and these will usually transfer to another school. Diploma school graduates generally work in the hospital setting.
- *Associate's degree in nursing:* at this level, you will attend community college for about 3 years and earn an associate's degree in nursing (ADN). You will earn approximately 60 hours of college credit in liberal arts, science, and nursing. These credits will usually transfer to a university should you decide to continue or return for a bachelor's degree. ADNs work primarily in hospitals and often in home health.
- *Bachelor's degree in nursing:* At this third level you'll go to a college for 4 years and earn a bachelor's degree in nursing (BSN). About half of the 120 to 140 credits you'll earn getting your BSN will be in liberal arts and science. The remainder will derive from nursing classes, including clinical practice, research, and courses related to the care of individuals, families, and populations. BSNs work in all health care settings.

ALL NURSES ARE NOT CREATED EQUAL

In each of the three undergraduate levels, once you have finished your degree program, you will be eligible to take the National Council License Examination for Registered Nursing (NCLEX). When you pass this test, you receive a nursing license giving you the legal right, under the requirements of your state's board of nursing, to practice as a registered nurse (RN). Therefore, even though all three levels bring you to the same end—an RN license—each route is different.

How do you decide which of these options to take? Ideally there should be just one choice, for the obvious reason that all these choices only add to the public's confusion about the nursing profession. But within the profession an argument over what is called *entry level to practice* has been going on for many years. Entry level to practice is simply the amount of basic nursing education, or degree requirement, that you need to take the NCLEX licensing examination and become an RN. The American Nurses Association, American Association of Colleges of Nursing, and other groups would like to see all RNs start out with a BSN degree. They argue that this requirement would help make nursing more professional and thereby improve its image. Why? Because a college degree is a basic requirement for other professions such as medicine, law, and teaching. Another important argument is that students need at least 4 years to learn the vast amount of basic information it takes to be a nurse.

However, advocates of the ADN degree say that their program makes nursing more accessible to a wider group of people: it costs less, takes less time, has less stringent admission requirements than BSN schools, and is more widely available. Both arguments have been discussed ad nauseam for years because no one can agree. Fortunately, nurses are starting to look beyond what has come to seem an unsolvable problem by focusing on what it takes to produce good nurses and how to prepare them to meet health care's changing needs. In this way, the entry level to practice issue may be solved. In Washington state all nursing education leaders have agreed to focus on the BSN or higher as the desirable RN degree.

NURSING EVOLUTION: SURVIVAL OF THE FITTEST?

Nursing as a profession with a structured training program has 137 years under its belt. Nurses were around a long time before this, but anything they learned then was learned on the job and not in school.

When Florence Nightingale returned from the Crimean War in the 1850s, she was determined to develop a training school for nurses. She believed that nurses needed specific knowledge about caring for the ill and careful instruction about moral character and the values of nursing. Around this time, most nurses were poor working women with little or no education who did what they had to to make the best living they could, including prostitution (the designation *nurse* was not based on educational or licensing requirements but merely on being paid to take care of the sick). Nightingale wanted to raise the status of nursing to that of a profession through structured, discipline-specific instruction and to counter the image of the nurse as illiterate and immoral by teaching students how to act orderly, ethically, and with decorum.

Nightingale achieved her goals by opening the first nurse's training school in 1860 at St. Thomas's Hospital in England. But during her time she was vehemently opposed by doctors, hospital managers, and even some nurses. They claimed that it was unnecessary for nurses to know anything about scientific theory, much less about the new so-called nursing theory. We know that education goes a long way toward helping people gain the power needed to change their circumstances, and it is thought that this was one of the major reasons Nightingale was opposed. Those who opposed Nightingale were not interested in seeing nurses, or women, upgrade their status, much less gain power. They preferred that women exercise any power they had in the home. Women were thought to be incapable of making decisions about anything else, since common belief held that women possessed inferior intellectual and physical capabilities.

For many years after this, nursing schools were located in hospitals. Students were trained by other nurses employed by that hospital. The students learned, but they also provided free labor. They cleaned bed linens, scrubbed floors, and washed dishes in exchange for the opportunity to learn nursing skills. The students worked long, hard hours, often strictly confined to the school premises and closely watched over by a head matron.

Those objecting to this strict training thought it unfair to make nursing students work so hard. Vigorously protesting the exploitation of the students, they were concerned that hospitals were not able to competently run both a school and their business without serious conflict of interest.

In 1909 the Rockefeller Foundation released a report recommending that nursing schools move out of the hospitals and into colleges or universities. This was a real boost for the advocates of college training. Howard University (a historically black university) established the first university-based nursing program in the U.S., although the University of Minnesota is generally credited with starting the program in 1909 and expanding that to the first BSN program in 1919.

Hospital schools continued to dominate nursing education until the 1960s, when community colleges with ADN programs gained popularity. The ADN programs were originally initiated because of a severe post-World War II nursing shortage: nurses were needed immediately. The community college programs were appealing because it took less time and money for a nurse to be trained and ready to work.

The nursing profession was very much against this change, but eventually a compromise was reached whereby the new ADNs would be designated technical nurses rather than professional RNs. They would provide care only under the direct supervision of a professional nurse. However, this plan never materialized. Dorothy D. Camilleri, former dean of the University of Illinois at Chicago School of Nursing, explained:

> The technical nurse would be under the direction of the professional nurse, a matter that would require appropriate licensing arrangements to be made by each state's board of nursing. These boards of nursing never did, however, create that distinction (a political move for sure) and neither did hospitals (most likely an economic move). Consequently, we have a single license for practice, with various paths to achieve it.

Today the American Nurses Association considers the ADN not a final nursing degree, but as a step on the ladder leading to a BSN. Nevertheless, although the ANA has made its recommendations, it is up to each state to pass legislation that would change the current system. This is the only way to change the entry level to practice issue to reflect the original intention of the 2-year degree programs and to create just one pathway to the RN degree: the BSN.

To understand nursing it is useful to remember that throughout the history of the profession it has been, and will continue to be, influenced by outside events. To be a nurse, then, you must have a grasp not only of health care but of politics, social issues, and economics. Dean Camilleri put it this way:

> The influence of an interacting web of societal events on decisions about nursing would be difficult to overestimate. Starting with politics, consider the occurrence of wars and their impact on available manpower, the need for health services for civilian and military populations, and the reorganization of male and female roles.... These are just examples of factors that, while external to nursing, form a powerful context for influencing decisions that are made about nursing.

FROM WHICH BRANCH SHOULD I SWING?

The world of health care today is complex and full of change, and experts in the field tell us to expect it to continue this way well into the 21st century. Nurses must be well equipped to deal with these changes. That's why it's important that you make the right decision about your education.

It is not only the number of years you study and the amount of information you acquire; it is also how you learn to think. You will need to know how to put together large amounts of information and make decisions using a plan of care that can, at times, spell life or death. Further, you must effectively communicate that plan, along with your rationale and results, to many different people.

With the variation in the quality of schools in our country, some high school graduates could perform this difficult task more easily than some college graduates.

However, the bottom line is that you should get the best education you can to meet the rigorous challenge of being a nurse. The decision about which type of program you choose is very important but, in most cases, not irrevocable. If you start in an ADN program, you can always switch to a BSN program.

In the past it didn't make much difference if you had an associate's degree, a diploma degree, or a bachelor's degree. A nursing job was a nursing job. Most nurses started as a staff nurse in a hospital doing direct patient care. After a year or two, depending on desire and ability, they moved to positions as head nurses, nursing supervisors, or directors of nursing.

These days, as in many other professions, jobs are becoming more complex, and the market has become more competitive. The old health care system is dying out, and a new system is being created before our eyes. Nurses need to know how to take care of their patients, but they must also be fluent in business, leadership, politics, management, and communication. Thus, although the change in health care brings rich opportunity, it also requires more knowledge and flexibility than was needed in the past. Protecting the quality of patient care and promoting health within this new system are the enormous tasks that nurses have before them.

What does this mean for you as a potential nurse trying to decide about whether to get an ADN or a BSN? A great deal. Nurses need a wider variety of skills than they used to—not just the kind of skills used for starting intravenous lines and reading monitors, but skills such as leadership; the ability to gather, analyze, and judge information used in clinical decision making; and the ability to communicate with all kinds of people in all kinds of situations. Clinical expertise is extremely important, but it must be more than the ability to carry out tasks. In many cases you will find that a prospective employer is looking for a nurse with a BSN to fill these roles.

For this very reason, Diane, RN, a student in one of my classes, was out of the running for a job she wanted. When I first met her, I asked her why she was returning to school for her BSN. She said it was an easy decision: "to get a promotion, make more money, and take on a new challenge." After working 12 years in the same job, she wanted to make a change. She had a special interest in patient teaching but was finding herself so busy being the manager of her unit that she didn't have the time anymore to work directly with the patients. She saw a job posting for a nurse educator in the new diabetes clinic, but it required a BSN and she had only an ADN. Shortly after losing this opportunity she returned to school to complete her BSN degree.

CHOOSING THE RIGHT PATH

I won't be discussing diploma programs, because they are becoming scarce. But if you are thinking about attending one, the ADN information will be most applicable for you. You can probably tell that I have a bias toward the BSN degree; this is because it's a given in our society that a college degree is the basic requirement for a profession and that nurses need, now more than ever, to get as much education as they can. When other health care professions such as physical therapy and pharmacy require a doctorate degree, I have to ask: Are these professions anymore complex than nursing? Do they require any more skill than nursing? The answer is NO.

Be that as it may, I do know that sometimes an ADN is the way to go. Let's look in more detail at the options.

Option 1: The BSN

You will begin at a 4-year college or university (or at a community college and transfer) and get a bachelor's degree in nursing. Many colleges offer a BSN degree just as they do a BA in English or a BS in zoology. With this degree, you will be ready if you choose to go on to graduate school.

Advantages
- *Competitiveness:* The National League for Nursing claims that the market is flooded with nurses with ADNs (42% of all RNs have an ADN). Although it takes longer to get a BSN, as a new graduate you will be more competitive. Some employers will even pay a BSN a higher salary. For example, in the Veterans Administration (VA) you will hit a ceiling on the pay scale, as well as on the promotion scale, with an ADN degree. Nurses who work for the VA often return to school to get better jobs with better pay.
- *Efficiency:* With a BSN you are ready to go to graduate school. If you have any desire to become a nurse practitioner, nurse midwife, anesthetist, educator, researcher, administrator, or other advanced practice specialist, you will need graduate school.
- *Comprehensiveness:* Why is this important? As a professional nurse you must have an excellent grasp of pathophysiology (diseases) and pharmacology (drugs), as well as an equally strong knowledge of psychology and sociology. The education you will receive from a general liberal arts curriculum will give you an advantage over an ADN or diploma nurse by virtue of the diversity of knowledge you will gain. Nurses work with all aspects of health, and this is why nursing is called a holistic health practice. Excellent communication skills are essential, and many colleges and universities require courses in speech and debate. This is crucial for the nurse today because nurses must be prepared to stand up and advocate not only for their patients but for the quality of health care and the profession of nursing itself. As such, you must be able to speak effectively and knowledgeably on a wide range of subjects.

Option 2: The ADN
You will attend a community college and get an ADN. Later, if you desire, you can return to school to earn your bachelor's degree and then go on to graduate school.

Advantages
- *A community college is less expensive and takes less time to complete.* You will be out of school and ready to work sooner than if you go for a BSN degree. Getting a bachelor's degree in nursing requires not only more time but more money (unless you get an ADN first and later return for a BSN, in which case it will cost you more time *and* more money.) Some nursing school advisers recommend that those with tight finances, little support, or a real need to get to work as soon as possible go to a community college.
- *Community colleges can be more user friendly.* For many students a community college is a great way to get started with their education. This can be especially true if you've been out of school for a while or prefer a smaller school. I've found that community colleges also tend to have more diversity in age and ethnicity of students and that classes are often smaller and more personal. When I first went back to college after dropping out of high school, I started at Seattle Community College, and I'm glad I did. I needed an environment that was friendly and flexible. If I had started at the University of Washington (where I did go later) and sat in a math class with 500 premed students and one teacher, I probably would have dropped out again.

- *You can work for a while and then, if you wish, return for a BSN.* Remember that you can always start at a community college and transfer to a university later on. There are programs available for nurses with ADN degrees who want to return to school for a BSN. These programs are designed to meet the needs of returning students. They often have fewer clinical requirements, and many have distant learning programs. In a distant learning program you don't have to live near the school, which is especially good if you live in a rural area. The university I work at has a program like this, and I teach students living over 200 miles away in the San Juan Islands, Montana, and Idaho. Students take the classes online and talk to me via e-mail or telephone.

THREE NEW NURSES MAKE THEIR WAY OUT OF THE PRIMORDIAL SOUP

The creation of a nurse is an interesting event. For a closer look at situations you might find yourself in that would influence your choice of ADN over BSN, I found three volunteers to share their early stories of becoming nurses.

"I Didn't Know I Wanted to Be a Nurse"

I worked in cardiac rehabilitation with a nurse, Mary, who lived in North Carolina and had a university degree in music. After several years of barely scratching out a living giving music lessons and playing in a band, she grew weary of not making much money.

One summer she happened to go to an area of Appalachia to help set up a music program for the community. What she saw there shocked her. She was not prepared for the rampant poverty and poor health. She said, "Here I was trying to set up a music program when these people didn't even have enough to eat. I knew that music was an important part of a good life, but it doesn't feed children or provide prenatal care to pregnant women."

After that Mary decided to go back to school to get a degree in nursing. This way, she could earn more money and provide a needed service. She went to evening classes for 1 year to pick up the science prerequisites she needed for admission to nursing school and then returned to the university, where she had earned her degree in music. In 2 more years she had her BSN. (Many universities offer this option as long as you meet the prerequisites for admission to their nursing program.)

Today Mary is a cardiac nurse and a musician. She plays music as a life-enriching activity, and she works as a nurse to earn money and serve humanity.

Mary's situation shows that if you already have a bachelor's degree in another area but have recently decided you want to be a nurse, you can go back to college and get a BSN as a second degree. Later, if you wish, you can go on to get a master's degree in nursing.

"I Can't Move to a University"

I was discussing the BSN versus ADN problem with Judy, a nurse I had worked with in the intensive coronary care unit. Judy told me that she wouldn't be where she was today if there hadn't been an ADN program where she lived (namely, one of those places without a university).

She knew she wanted to be a nurse, but at the time she didn't have the option of going away to school, because she couldn't afford it. She enrolled in a local ADN program, got her degree, and worked in a small community hospital for several years. Then she moved to a larger city, where she returned to school for her BSN while working in the cardiac intensive care unit of a large hospital. Eventually she went on for her master's degree, just because she loved school so much, and got a job teaching nursing students while she worked on her PhD. If Judy had not had the opportunity to attend an ADN program and consequently had never become a nurse, it would have been a serious loss for the nursing profession. She is one of the most caring nurses I know, she is great with her students and her patients, and she projects the kind of intelligence and professionalism that make her a credit to nursing.

If there are no colleges where you live that offer BSN degrees and you want to be a nurse, check with a local librarian for information from neighboring schools. Some may have distant learning programs. These are usually for ADNs going on for a BSN or for graduate students, but check anyway so you know what is available.

"I'm Divorced, and I Have to Get a Job Now!"

When Jerry, whose wife had been working full time while he stayed home taking care of their kids, and his wife divorced, he was broke. It had been 3 years since he had held a job. Jerry needed to work, but he wanted a job that would pay above minimum wage and have opportunities for advancement. He would have liked to go to a university, but he couldn't afford to spend the time or the money. So he enrolled in a community college and earned his ADN. After working in a community hospital for 2 years as a staff nurse, he was promoted to a managerial position in the Emergency Department.

Jerry eventually returned to graduate school to earn a master's degree as a nurse anesthetist. "If I had not gone to the community college," he says, "I would never be where I am today."

If you need a job as soon as possible and if waiting to get into school, much less having it take 4 years to get a degree is not an option, an ADN program can be a stepping-stone to getting a BSN later, when your circumstances allow.

BSN OR ADN: WHERE YOU MIGHT BE WORKING

The National League for Nursing claims that new ADNs are most likely to find work in care settings such as hospitals and nursing homes. According to the American Association of Colleges of Nursing, new BSN graduates should be prepared to work in all settings, including community and public health and ambulatory settings such as clinics.

The most recent statistics show that 78% of ADNs work in hospitals compared with 88.8% of BSNs. Nursing homes have 14.4% of the ADNs on their workforce with only 5.2% of the BSNs. Community or public health is where 5.1% of ADNs and 4.6% of BSNs are working. Although nursing organizations are telling us that BSNs are more likely than ADNs to work outside of the hospital, the statistics show that this is not currently the case.

Table 5-1 provides a brief comparison of each type of program—ADN and BSN.

TAKING IT ONE STEP AT A TIME

The nursing adviser at Washington State University told me that she looks at nursing education as occurring in steps. The BSN is the preferred degree, but you can start with an ADN and work from there. The master's degree and doctoral degree come next. With each step you add flexibility, the ability to get more interesting jobs, and the opportunity to become an entrepreneur with your own business.

Just about every nurse I've read about or talked to recommends that, if at all possible, you get a BSN degree first. Nurses who have ADN degrees agree. Judy advises,

TABLE 5-1	Outline of ADN and BSN Programs	
Program Characteristic	**ADN**	**BSN**
Where?	Community and junior colleges	Colleges or universities
How long?	2-3 years of full-time study; ≈60 credit hours	4 years of full-time study; ≈120 credit hours
Prerequisites?	High school or equivalent degree; varying GPAs for admission	High school or equivalent degree; varying GPAs between 2.5 to 3.0 for admission*
Basic courses?	≈1/3: General education classes ≈2/3: Biological and social sciences classes	≈1/3: General education classes ≈2/3: Biological and social sciences classes
Nursing courses?	Adult and child health Legal and ethical issues Psychiatric and mental health Professional practice	Same as ADN, *plus* community and public health management Research and statistics Leadership

ADN, Associate's degree in nursing; BSN, bachelor's degree in nursing.
*See the section on applications in Chapter 6.

"If you can, just go ahead and get the BSN. It will save you time later." Likewise, Jerry said, "I would have gone for my BSN right off if I had known I wanted to do anything besides work as a staff nurse. Now I want to become a nurse anesthetist and need to get my master's degree."

Over the years both types of nurses can gain equivalent knowledge, but the BSN is more likely to be able to make the jump into new health care opportunities and move up the career ladder.

There are many positions in health care to be filled. But if you want to work in a more advanced role or practice more independently, I strongly advise that you start with a college BSN degree and then plan on getting a graduate degree. (See Appendix A for additional information and career resources.)

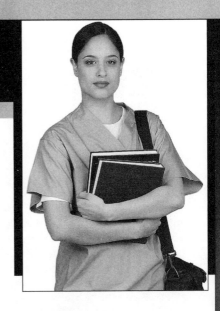

Invasive Procedures: Getting into School

THIS WON'T HURT A BIT: MATH AND SCIENCE

Any degree you choose, be it nursing, engineering, law, or some other field, requires you to take specific courses called prerequisites before you begin advanced courses in that major. Prerequisites for a bachelor's degree in nursing (BSN) vary somewhat from school to school but usually include the following:

- organic chemistry
- inorganic chemistry
- biochemistry
- microbiology
- biologic science
- anatomy
- physiology
- statistics
- nutrition
- human development

Some schools are omitting microbiology as a prerequisite for the major, but I strongly suggest that you take it if you can because, with antibiotic resistance and viral diseases on the rise, this content is relevant and worth understanding. The associate's degree in nursing (ADN) prerequisites are less stringent and are sometimes taken in the first year of the program or intermixed with the nursing courses. Science courses such as chemistry, statistics, and microbiology usually are not required.

At Washington State University students take all the prerequisites in the first and second years of college and the nursing courses in the third and fourth years. Other schools integrate the courses over the 4 years.

If you are returning to school with previous college credits, you will want to have them evaluated for transfer credit. For instance, if you took a chemistry class at another school, your new school will let you know if they will count that class for your chemistry requirement. Some schools will not accept transfer credit for classes taken more than 5 to 10 years ago. This, too, varies widely from school to school.

If you want to attend a BSN program such as the one at Washington State University, you have to take the prerequisites before you can be admitted to the nursing school. At other schools you can take them while you are there. ADN students who wish to enter a BSN program can usually transfer many of their ADN course credits.

Many students are afraid of taking science courses. Nancy, RN, confided that, when she decided to return to school after raising her two children, the thought of taking chemistry terrified her. All she could think of was how much she had hated high school chemistry. When she returned to school, the first prenursing class she took was biology. Her grade was a C. She said, "I thanked God every day for that C."

She knew that, if she were to continue in school with any success, she would have to find a way to get through chemistry. She explained, "Chemistry was like traveling to a foreign land with a foreign language. I couldn't understand any of it." So she went to her school's learning center and found a tutor who was a graduate student in chemistry. For the first 2 months of the semester she met with him after every class to review the material. Her final grade in organic chemistry was an A.

By working with the tutor, she learned how to review on her own or with other students and went on to receive A's in all her prerequisite nursing school classes. She advises all students who are uneasy about science courses to visit their school learning center and find out who, or what, is available to help them. She explained,

"If you want to be a nurse but are afraid of science or math, you'll have to be very determined. Don't let embarrassment keep you from asking for help."

Many people have a difficult time with math and science courses because they are afraid of them. Overcoming that fear by getting extra help may be all you need to succeed. Once you get past the fear factor, like Nancy, you can do very well.

WHY ME? WHY SCIENCE? WHY MATH?

If you don't have a realistic view of what nurses do, these are questions you might be asking. For example, some students who say they love babies and just want a job working with babies, ask, "Would nursing be a way to do that?" and "Why do I need science to work with babies?" Let's look at this a little further.

Imagine you are a labor and delivery nurse and your patient has just had a baby. Both the baby and the mother have developed an infection. They are going to need an intravenous (IV) antibiotic, and it is your job to give it to them. What are you going to do?

First, the IV will probably come premixed from the pharmacy. It will tell you the correct rate at which to run the medication to get the correct dose of antibiotic you want. You follow the instructions, but the pharmacy made a mistake, and you've just unwittingly given the baby the wrong dose, with potentially catastrophic results.

Now let's run through that example again. In nursing school you took all those math and science prerequisites and learned how to calculate dosages. Therefore you can easily figure out at how many milliliters you should run the IV in order to give the correct number of micrograms of antibiotic. You also know from biochemistry that a chemical reaction of the antibiotic occurs in the kidneys. So you are very careful not to give the drug incorrectly because you could cause kidney damage in either of your patients.

You receive the drug from the pharmacy, and this time you check it by recalculating the equation. Noticing the mistake, you call the pharmacy, and they correct it and send you another. You recheck it again, and this time it is right. You give the right dose of the drug to the baby. You also think about possible side effects and what you will need to keep track of for both the mother and the baby. In the end mother and baby are happy and healthy and give you a big thank-you as they leave the hospital for home.

This example is not intended to imply that pharmacists often make mistakes. But everyone makes mistakes. Nurses make mistakes. Doctors make mistakes. And your job, along with the rest of the health care team, is to do your best to prevent them. A strong background in science and math is crucial to this end. Science is paramount in giving you the skills you need to provide safe, rational, and effective nursing care. Just as a pilot must understand aerodynamics or why the plane stays in the air, so nurses need to understand all the things that keep people alive and healthy because people's lives are in their hands, too.

Science teaches you how to think critically and observe and how to reason and problem solve. Ask any nurse and the nurse will tell you that she or he uses these skills every day. You must remember, too, that nurses work with the whole person. They take care of their bodies and their minds; science teaches you about how the mind works, too.

If you deal with psychiatric problems, and almost all nurses do, no matter what area they work in, you need science to help you understand treatments and to think about things such as the effect sleep deprivation or poor nutrition might have on a patient's behavior.

The humanities are equally important. By taking psychology and sociology courses you will learn theories and principles that will guide you in working with people in all kinds of situations. This is what nurses do. They apply the knowledge learned in school, on the job, and in continuing education classes to real-life situations. If you want to do safe, high-quality work, you must be well educated.

The Emergency Department (ED) is a good place to observe nurses using many different kinds of skills. To act and think quickly ED nurses need to understand many physiologic and psychologic principles. Barb, an ED nurse, told me that one day she saw a woman who had come in four or five times in 1 month because she kept falling down. Without a science background, Barb might have told her to go home and rest.

By the time Barb saw her, the woman had had three CT scans, which are very expensive procedures, to determine the cause of her falls. Barb's scientific background had taught her skills of observation and deduction. She found out through questioning and reading her chart that the woman wasn't dizzy and didn't have any arrhythmias (heartbeat irregularities). After she had still more inconclusive tests, Barb wondered if there was some nonmedical cause for her falls. As she was helping her get dressed to go home, using her acute observation skills, she noticed that she had worn the heel off her shoe and that she was trying to walk around on plastic. It turns out that she just needed a new pair of shoes. Barb said, "Those are the things that you do as a nurse. The hospital has spent $11,000 on needless tests, and all she needed was a new pair of shoes."

I've given you some relatively simple examples (believe me, they can get much more complex) to illustrate the point that science and math are a necessary component of nursing. Thus, while a love of babies is definitely not a reason in itself to go into nursing, it can be a good place to start if you are prepared to back it up with a strong background in science.

APPLYING TO SCHOOL: FOR EXTERNAL USE ONLY

The application process is straightforward, but start early! For instance, applications for admittance to the fall nursing class may be due as early as January. Your school adviser can help you get through it. You will begin applying to nursing school at least one semester before you will start. If you are still taking prerequisites at that time, you may get a conditional acceptance, which means that you are accepted to nursing school assuming you complete and pass your current courses. You should expect to compete with other students for admission to most nursing programs. In the fall of 2006, Washington State University College of Nursing had 341 applicants. Of those, 230 were interviewed, and 130 admitted.

Find out what the waiting list is like for the school you want to attend. Many schools, especially universities, will look carefully at your grade point average (GPA), especially in the prerequisite courses; your ability to express yourself in writing; and the reasons you want to become a nurse. GPA can be a determining factor when it comes to who gets accepted to nursing school in the first round and who has to wait or who doesn't get in at all. Some advisers say their schools require a 2.5 GPA, but you are less likely to be accepted unless you have a 3.0 or higher GPA. Some say that a 3.5 GPA or higher is pretty much the norm for admission. Your best bet is to ask the nursing schools you wish to apply to what GPA they consider to be the most competitive.

When I went to nursing school, I had a 3.7 GPA and was accepted in the first round. I did well in science, which helped my GPA a great deal. Luckily I loved science, which was probably because I grew up in a family that was not science-oriented. My father was a librarian, and my mother an English major. Books were our world. Science was for people who worked in smelly, poorly lit laboratories on sunny days or who stayed up all night drinking bad coffee in gloomy observatories while peering through a telescope.

When I took my first science class in community college, I felt like a rebel, like I was blazing a new trail. Since I had dropped out of high school, the last time I took science was eighth-grade. The first class I took in community college was a plant identification course in which I discovered in great detail the interesting anatomy of plants. Doing well in that class, I was secretly thrilled. I thought, if I can do this, why not try another one? I went on to take astronomy, chemistry, and physics. It opened up a whole new world to me. I loved studying isomers, nebulas, and black holes. The idea of an invisible world where mirror images of molecules existed intrigued me as if it was a special kind of magic.

That was the beginning of my nursing career. I liked science, and it liked me; but, if you are more like Nancy, who was petrified of chemistry, take heart. With support and guidance from your school, family, or friends, you can make it. Make sure you work hard, get help, and keep your GPA as high as possible. However, if you do fall short of the mark, you could still become a nurse. You just might be on a waiting list before you are finally accepted. Many nursing schools are also interviewing prospective students. Check with an advisor to learn about preparing for an interview.

HOW MUCH WILL THIS TORTURE COST?

The price of school varies, depending on where it is located, whether it is a private or public school, and, if public, whether you must pay resident or nonresident tuition. The National League for Nursing reports that a bachelor's degree in nursing can cost anywhere from $3,000 to $10,000 a year; community college can cost $1,600 to $7,000 per year; and diploma programs average $3,500 per year.

These averages represent tuition only and do not include fees, books, uniforms, or living expenses. (Books alone can cost $400 a year.) In addition, many schools require application, laboratory, and graduation fees. Take time to figure out how much money you will need. Start with tuition; add fees and books, rent and food, transportation, and uniforms and other special equipment such as a stethoscope. This will give you a good idea of how much nursing school will cost. The reference section of almost any library contains books that will help you estimate the cost of your nursing education. Also refer to *Peterson's Nursing Programs 2005*, 10th revised edition (2004, Peterson's Guides/Thomson Learning), published in cooperation with the American Association of Colleges of Nursing; and The National League for Nursing's *A Guide to State-Approved Schools of Nursing RN*, now in its 57th edition (2006) Both provide information about the cost of individual schools and financial aid.

SOMEONE IS GOING TO PAY FOR THIS!

Money is available through grants, scholarships, and loans; be creative and check out all your options. Your school will have a financial aid officer to talk to, but he or she may not always know every available opportunity. You must take some of the responsibility yourself. Contact the head of the nursing department and ask for specifics on grants, loans, and assistantships. Many community groups can help you through school. Talk to local business and professional groups. Start with the

American Nurses Association and work down to your state association and your local district association. Most offer scholarships or grants (money you don't have to pay back).

The local nurses association where I live offers several $500 scholarships per year to nursing students. Numerous other nursing organizations do the same. Scholarship applications often require you to write a short essay on health care or the nursing profession, a task that many people would rather not do. But you should. Five hundred dollars may not pay for school, but every $500 helps. So seek out all your possibilities and spend the time filling out the applications.

When Marta was in graduate school to become a family nurse practitioner, she calculated that it took 4 hours to complete an application for a $500 scholarship. She received the award and figured that at $125 per hour, the application process wasn't so bad after all. She was awarded the scholarship based on her merit as a student, but the probability of her getting the award was greatly increased by the fact that few other students applied, possibly daunted by the application process itself. Take the time to search out these opportunities and, like Jennifer, who was working full-time and going to school full-time, take the time to meticulously fill out the applications while thinking about the end results.

Go to your library and check out a book called *Scholarships and Loans for Nursing Education* (which includes loans for specialty areas, ADN, BSN, minorities, and graduate students); get a publication from the U.S. Department of Education called *Funding Education Beyond High School: the Guide to Federal Student Aid*, http://studentaid.ed.gov/students/publications/student_guide/index.html; or call 1-800 4-FED-AID (1-800-433-3243). One excellent, easy-to-use book is *Loans and Grants From Uncle Sam: Am I Eligible and for How Much?* by Anna Leider, now in its 13th edition (2005, Octameron Associates). This book tells you in simple language what types of loans are available and how to determine if you are eligible for them; it also discusses repayment options and covers loans specifically for health professions. The publications are updated every 1 to 2 years and will help with all sorts of creative money sources. You can also ask the reference librarian for help. If you feel shy, remember that his or her job is to help you find the information you need. What may seem a tedious task to you is a librarian's bread and butter, perhaps even their passion. If you are from a particular ethnic group or culture, check with local organizations. For instance, the Hispanic Business Leaders Association, your Tribal council or other group may offer generous scholarships well worth pursuing.

And don't forget about the military, who offer scholarships in return for a specified amount of time in their service. Besides the Army, Navy, and Air Force, there are other branches you can join such as the Public Health Services, where you usually work in an underserved area after you graduate. (Exact definitions for underserved areas vary, but in general the term refers to geographic regions where there are not enough health care providers for the population.)

A final word about money: it is worth your while to consider all options for schooling, even if you think you can't afford them; sometimes spending more will bring you greater success in your education. Although Marta started graduate studies at a state school because it cost the least amount of money, after she completed a class or two she transferred to a private school. The private school Marta transferred to cost more money, but to her it was worth it. She said:

> The general atmosphere among the students at the state school was extremely competitive, and the faculty seemed unsupportive. I just didn't see the reason for

subjecting myself to that kind of agony. The private school was much better. I didn't like spending all the money—but it was worth it. There was a strong sense of camaraderie among the students that really made a difference to me and helped me to get through the program. Besides, the program was more flexible for me as a working nurse.

It is always tempting to pay the least amount possible when spending money, even if quality is sacrificed. On the other hand, spending loads of money on an expensive school doesn't guarantee you'll get a better education. The University of Washington in Seattle is ranked as one of the top nursing schools in the country, yet it costs less than many other schools.

Marta mentions flexibility (being able to take classes in the evening, on weekends, or all in only 1 day a week) as a factor in her decision. This is especially important if you are trying to work and go to school at the same time. The National League for Nursing says that 80% of all nursing students work part-time while they are attending school compared with only 15% of all other students.

OVER MY DEAD BODY AND OTHER AREAS OF SPECIAL INTEREST

On career day, high school students can be counted on to ask me, "Have you ever seen a dead body?" While this may be of interest, it is not my special interest. Nursing has many specialty areas—pediatrics, obstetrics, oncology, community, and mental health, to name just a few. If you already know what specialty area you want to work in and you can take time to look at different schools (if you aren't restricted to what is in your immediate area), ask questions about the professors' areas of expertise. Although it is true that most nursing curriculums are similar, it is also true that each school has its own specialty (for example, research, obstetrics, or cardiac care). You can interview a prospective school to see if it meets your needs in exactly the same way the school personnel interview you to see if you meet theirs. This is your education, your money, and your time; in fact, it is your life. If you haven't decided on an area of specialization (and most students haven't), there are other ways to make the decision about which school to attend. Interview past and present students (ask the school's admissions office for names and numbers if you don't know anyone). You can also go to the library and read about the school using a reference book such as the previously mentioned A Guide to State-Approved Schools of Nursing RN and by asking the librarian to help you find information about what a specific school has to offer you.

Remember that you are the customer in this situation, and, although some schools are very picky about whom they admit, they need you in order to stay in business. You have a right to ask them questions to find out what they are like before you sign on the dotted line on the enrollment form and give them your money. Once you have decided to which degree interests you (an ADN or BSN), start researching the actual schools. Find a program that's right for you academically, socially, financially, and geographically.

Chapter

7

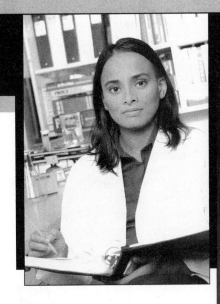

Going to School

Beginning school is a momentous time in anyone's life (although starting your first intravenous (IV) line successfully is also pretty momentous—it is a real thrill.) Whether you are straight out of high school, continuing in college, or returning to school after an absence, you can be absolutely sure that you are doing something of consequence. Becoming a nurse is difficult but extremely rewarding. There is so much to learn in school, but school is really just the beginning because nursing is a career for those who want to be lifelong learners.

Of course, at times during your school experience you will think that there is too much to learn. I remember studying for tests and feeling certain that I couldn't possibly remember one more piece of information, much less bring it back up at test time. Or worse, I had a vision of standing at a patient's bedside with my instructor ready to observe me perform a procedure I had diligently practiced the evening before and forgetting everything—standing there, mind blank, wondering: why am I here? At times you are bound to feel there is just too much to learn, but years later I still remember information I learned in school and then rarely used again, such as how to assess for tactile fremitus or diaphragmatic excursion. So have faith in the power of your memory: it will surprise you.

OPEN MIND IS NOT LEAKY MIND

Australian nurse Elizabeth Kenny tells us that some minds remain open only long enough for the truth to enter and to "pass on through by way of a ready exit without pausing anywhere along the route." The goal in nursing school is to keep your mind open not only long enough for new information and ideas to enter, but for you to actually soak them up—before they run back out.

While doing research for this book, I came upon the American Association of Colleges of Nursing (AACN) list of priorities for a bachelor's degree in nursing (BSN) education. I include them below to let you see your future education through your professor's eyes since it covers much of what you will learn in school:

1. Critical thinking
2. Ethical decision making
3. Coordination of care
4. Critical self-assessment

In addition to learning nursing's role in providing high-quality care, students should learn about the development of healthy lifestyles and how to solve problems in health care. The AACN recommends schools that include the following areas in their curriculums:

- Chronic conditions such as cardiovascular disease, cancer, and mental illness
- Infectious diseases, particularly HIV infection, sexually transmitted diseases, and tuberculosis
- Acute conditions such as accidental injuries/trauma
- Nutrition
- Family planning
- Maternal-infant health
- Substance abuse prevention
- Environmental and occupational health
- Geriatric health
- Prevention of family and social violence

Following is a listing of additional areas you should look for in a nursing school's curriculum:

- Economics of health care, including reimbursement
- Legal principles

- Political and social action
- Disaster preparedness
- International and global health experiences

There is much to learn, but the school you attend will also teach you how to understand, analyze, and incorporate that knowledge so you can use it when you become a registered nurse (RN).

REARRANGING AND SEWING BACK UP

You will be a different person when you graduate as a nurse. Not because nursing school brings on some kind of mysterious personality transformation, but because you will have begun to think about things in a different way. Nurses have a special way of thinking, and this is part of what you will be learning in school.

Of course, you will learn many facts such as the pH of blood and the signs and symptoms of various drug reactions. You will also learn many technical skills such as how to insert nasogastric tubes, attach a heart monitor, and take a blood pressure; and you will spend endless hours reading about diseases, surgical procedures, psychology, family dynamics, community systems, spirituality, and ethics. But, overall, what you will really begin to learn is how to think and how to problem solve.

When I first worked in cardiac intensive care, I was on the night shift, 11 PM to 7 AM. The other nurses and I used to go to a cafe after work. We would sit around a big table watching the morning customers as they came in for their shots of espresso. If we'd see a man whose face was stiff on the left side, we'd think to ourselves that he probably had a stroke. But when we noticed that his left arm was all right, we thought he might have Bell's palsy. We'd see a woman who seemed short of breath and had a round, puffy face; skin that was dry and thin; and very thin legs. She was probably on steroids for lung disease.

This kind of observation can be hard for nonnurses to understand, but it is a habit that almost all nurses develop; it becomes automatic. The thinking process learned in school and with experience on the job includes knowing how to gather clues, at times even subconsciously (often called intuition), put them together in a logical pattern, and form a hypothesis.

In the café, forming hypotheses was as far as we got. In our jobs the next step would have been to test our ideas. We'd listen to the woman's lungs, take a medication history, and check her blood sugar. The man would get a neurologic examination and have a health history taken. With this information a bigger picture would be formed; and more hypotheses developed, tested, and evaluated. This is what you learn in nursing school. It is a complicated process and one that nurse researchers like Patricia Benner have studied for years.

Benner studies nurses while they are doing their work, noting what they do and asking them why they do it. She was the first person to map out the complexity of nurses' thinking and how the complexity of that thinking was related to their level of expertise. In her model, when you graduate from nursing school, you are a novice; you have beginner's mind. So you see, nursing school is really just a start. When you are there, you should study hard and use the opportunity to start learning how to think like a nurse.

In case I haven't painted the picture clearly, let me say that nursing school can be stressful. You may feel more pressure to learn the technical skills of nursing, such as giving injections and starting IVs, than you will to learn the theories behind those skills. At school you will probably get a checklist of technical skills you will be expected to learn. It is so easy to become obsessed with checking these off and comparing your list with those of other students that the theories and principles underlying these skills are lost.

Don't let that happen, though, because this reasoning and inquiry (which at the time may seem trivial compared with the tubes, monitors, and medications) are lifesavers. They are what differentiate an average nurse from an excellent nurse. In school you will think that you don't have time to do and learn it all. And, of course, you probably don't, but I strongly advise you to try to put the technical skills in perspective. It may seem like the skills are the most important part of nursing, but trust me and the thousands of other nurses who would tell you the same thing— they are not. Thinking and problem solving are the foundation of nursing. If that foundation is weak, all the rest of the fancy trim will crumble into mediocrity and lost opportunity; worst of all, you will be an unsafe nurse.

WAKE UP, IT'S NOT OVER YET: THE NCLEX®

When you graduate from nursing school you should definitely celebrate the occasion. It is a real milestone and not one to be passed over lightly. However, you're not quite finished—you still have to take the licensing examination, the National Certifying Licensure Examination, or NCLEX, so that you can call yourself a registered nurse. Before you take and pass the exam your title will not be RN. To apply to take the exam, your nursing degree must be completed. This degree, either BSN, or ADN, allows you to sit for the exam. Many students take a NCLEX course to prepare for the exam from Kaplan (www.kaplan.com), or from their own school. In terms of your employability, you will need to pass the exam before you begin practicing. But, many students are looking for positions, and even accepting them, before they take and pass the NCLEX. So, you may have a position all lined up, but you will have to wait until you pass the exam to begin working as an RN. You will find out much more about this process once you are in nursing school. If you can't wait that long and want to know more, you can go to the Kaplan website.

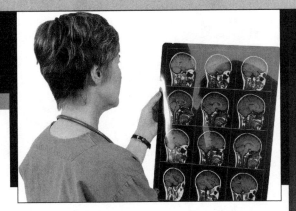

Need a Brain Transplant?

Try Graduate School

THE FUTURE IS USING YOUR BRAIN

One trend occurring in health care today involves managing the care of individual patients or populations of patients to ensure that it is efficient and consistent. This can result in fewer episodes of acute illness because managers are catching potential problems before they lead to crises. Nurses with graduate degrees (master's or doctorate's) who become advanced practice nurses are well trained to provide this kind of care. Furthermore, the Division of Nursing of the Health Resources and Services Administration (HRSA 2006) tells us that 8.3% of all RNs have an advanced practice degree. Of these 51% are nurse practitioners, 24% clinical nurse specialists, 13% certified nurse anesthetists, and 4% nurse midwives. To become an advanced practice nurse (APN), you must get a graduate degree. For a master's degree this requires about 2 years of full-time study. The cost varies, depending on the school. Graduate tuition is often more expensive than undergraduate tuition, but scholarships and assistantships are available.

Grade point averages (GPAs) also play a bigger role in admissions. It is not unusual for a 3.0 GPA to be the minimum requirement. Courses in graduate school are divided into two areas, core and specialty. The core courses focus on research, clinical, and leadership skills; and the specialty courses focus on the area of your major. If you were becoming a nurse practitioner (NP), you would take courses such as physical assessment and many, many hours of clinical experience.

SPECIALTY DU JOUR: ADVANCED PRACTICE

APNs are distinguished by specialty area, such as a clinical nurse specialist or an NP. Other APNs with graduate degrees who work with patients indirectly include nurse administrators or educators (although there is a new degree specialty called a clinical nurse leader who is a manager who specializes in clinical care).

Changes that are occurring regarding regulation of APNs include the definition of APN and what APNs are called. The four types of APNs currently regulated by most states are: nurse midwife, clinical nurse specialist, nurse anesthetist, and NP (which is broken down into further specialties). For example, if want to be an NP, you must have a master's degree in nursing from a school that grants a degree in that specialty. But first you will have to decide what kind of NP you'd like to be: adult, family, women's health, mental health, pediatric, neonatal, or geriatric, to name just a few.

State regulation as an APN generally means that you have prescriptive authority. There is a movement among some state board's of nursing to no longer allow clinical nurse specialists to be licensed as APNs, even though they are still advanced practice nurses. Confusing? You will need to go to the National Boards of Nursing and the American Association of Nursing to understand more about the issues. But, in a nutshell, the controversy has to do with who is defining nursing practice: the state regulating board or the nurses' professional organization.

Another big change is a new degree program for NPs called a Doctorate in Nursing Practice, or the DNP. By the year 2015 all NPs will have to have this degree. The DNP program would continue immediately after the bachelor's degree in nursing (BSN) program; a master's degree would not be required. As with all things in nursing, there is also debate about the formation of this new degree but you don't have to worry about that now.

Currently, if you know you'd like to work in a specific area (for example, women's health), you'd get your master's degree from a school with an NP program in women's health. But if you prefer something more diverse, the family NP degree is the most general of these degrees, allowing you to work with people of all ages in many different settings.

Another example of an APN degree is in anesthesia, which also requires a master's degree from a school with a nurse anesthetist program. There are fewer of these than other APN programs, and they can be very competitive; but the need for nurse anesthetists is growing, and the salary is excellent.

Table 8-1 shows various specialty areas for APNs, including what they do, where they do it, and with whom they work. In light of the anticipated shortage of APNs, obtaining your APN degree is a wise career path to consider. There are other graduate degrees in nursing. Health administration and policy is one; community health is another.

STOP THE TRANSPLANT: MY CRANIUM'S TOO SMALL

When I went to graduate school, I specialized in education. I probably will regret saying this, but this came about a bit by accident; and if my current employers happen to read this, let me say that it turned out to be a positive accident, because I love teaching. It's okay to be worried at this point about what you are going to do with your life, much less with what area of nursing you want to go into; just keep an open mind.

When I first went to nursing school, my goal was to become an NP. When I graduated with my BSN, I initially wanted to work in pediatrics, but there were no jobs. So I tried the neonatal intensive care unit, but during the interview I decided I wasn't too keen on the people there. Then I heard of a friend of a friend who was a nurse in cardiac care. She loved her job, she loved her manager, and they had openings on the night shift. And this is how I got into cardiac nursing. There were no big deliberations, no flashes of light, no lifelong goal to work in this particular place—just an opening, a good boss, and a few friends.

I thought, "I'll work here for a year, and then I'll be an expert cardiac nurse. Then I'll return to school." After my first year on the job, though, I saw quite plainly that I was no expert—not even close. During my first annual evaluation I burst into tears because I didn't get superior marks in all areas. The manager looked at me quizzically and said, "What did you expect after only 1 year? You've got years of learning ahead."

I dried my tears, took my wounded ego by the hand, and really applied myself to learning the job of cardiac nurse. This took about 10 years, at which time I again thought about school, but I wasn't sure what I wanted to do. The NP idea wasn't as appealing as it had been, and I thought, "Why go to graduate school and spend a lot of time and money if I don't know what I want to do?" I forgot that I never really knew what I wanted to do to begin with. Four years later, when I remembered that I never really knew, I decided to go to graduate school anyway, thinking that maybe I'd make a discovery there; maybe some lucky event would come my way.

My first year in graduate school was fine because I took only the required core courses; no decisions about specializing were necessary. But eventually I had to decide. I thought about the family NP program; and, because all my friends at school were doing it, I seriously considered it. I asked myself, "Do you want a job in a clinic seeing patients, including children, all day?" The answer was a clear no, because that was not the kind of work that interested me most. I wanted to spend more time teaching, writing, and perhaps doing research. And I could have done these things as an NP, but I wanted to spend my time in school focusing on my areas of interest.

TABLE 8-1	Comparison of Specialties for Advanced Practice Nurses		
Advanced Practice Nurse	**Application of Advanced Knowledge and Skills**	**Patient Population Served**	**Practice Settings**
Certified midwife	Well-women health care Management of pregnancy, childbirth, antepartum, and postpartum care Health promotion	Childbearing women	Homes Hospitals Birthing centers Ambulatory care
Clinical nurse specialist	Management of complex patient health care problems in various clinical specialty areas through direct care, consultation, research, education, and administration	Individuals with physical or psychiatric illness and disability Maternal and child health problems	Hospitals Ambulatory care Community care Home health rehabilitation
Nurse anesthetist	Preoperative assessment Administration of anesthesia Recovery	Individuals in all age-groups who are undergoing surgical procedures	Hospital operating rooms Ambulatory care Surgical settings
Nurse practitioner	Management of a wide range of health problems through physical examination, treatment, and family/patient education and counseling Primary care Health promotion	Individuals and families Women, infants, and children Elderly adults and others	Primary care Long-term care Ambulatory care Community care Hospitals

Data from the American Association of Colleges of Nursing (AACN): *Your nursing career: a look at the facts*. Washington, DC, March 10, 2004, AACN. Retrieved July 10, 2006, from www.aacn.nche.edu/Education/nurse_ed/career.htm.

So what next? I had to think about what I liked most in nursing, and the answer to that was teaching. I loved patient teaching. So I specialized in education. Now I teach nursing students in a university, and I teach patients in a cardiac rehabilitation program. For me, it's the best of all worlds. I "lucked out" by allowing myself room to not know what I wanted to do.

Of course, not everyone operates the way I do; so try the following exercise to help you clarify your interests. It is similar to your Pros and Cons list: on a piece of paper make two columns. In column A list all the things that interest you, and in column B the things that definitely do not interest you. This will help you start thinking about what you might like to do and help you begin to plan for school. Remember, though, your interests are likely to change as time goes by; so let your list be flexible and don't box yourself in.

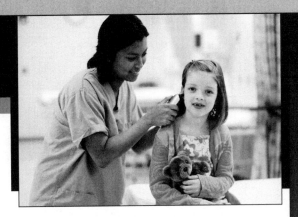

The Insider's Scoop
on Job Opportunities

Nursing is the fastest growing health care profession, and the need for nurses in all areas of practice will continue. Finding a job once you finish nursing school is not a problem, but you need to be prepared to understand what you want and how to get it. This chapter focuses on employment options.

WATCH OUT FOR THAT TREE!

Nursing is notorious for job market swings. For example, when I graduated from nursing school in the early 1980s, there were plenty of jobs because the economy was doing well and, with new technologies and hospital services, health care was booming. By the end of the 1980s, the boom peaked, hospitals were filled to capacity, and there were not enough nurses to take care of all the patients. New graduates were beginning their first nursing jobs on the day shift—usually the most coveted and most difficult shift to obtain—and, on top of that, getting sign-on cash bonuses. Then in the late 1990s the pendulum swung in the other direction, and many new graduates worried about finding a job of any kind, on any shift. However, a new kind of nursing shortage is now in full swing.

Health care economics are changing. Basically the system that we've grown up with is transforming. One driving force is money; and, in an attempt to curb costs, hospitals and other health care businesses are trying to be more efficient. The time a patient spends in the hospital costs the health care system a lot of money. Imelda, a retired nurse, remembers when patients were admitted to the hospital for a "rest," as if the hospital were a hotel. Insurance companies paid the cost of any stay sanctioned by the doctor, no matter what the reason or for how long. Today a person has to be very sick to be admitted and he or she stays a much shorter time. Altogether this means that care is more complex.

Research is beginning to show that hospitals with the lowest ratio of registered nurses (RNs) to patients have the highest numbers of patient complications, readmissions, and employee injuries. Nurse staffing levels are directly tied to safety and quality of care. I read a letter to the editor in the journal *American Nurse* about an RN working in a hospital who at the end of a shift asked a nursing aide about the results of a routine morning blood sugar check of patient with diabetes. The level was very low. When the nurse asked him why he hadn't reported it earlier, he said, "The patient was fine. He was sleeping peacefully." Understanding that what appeared to be peaceful sleep could be loss of consciousness due to low blood sugar, the nurse ran to the room.

Nurses have always been concerned with the quality of patient care, and they want to make sure that quality is not sacrificed in an attempt to save money; rather, they want to ensure that quality care is given while money is saved. It is not wise to blindly embrace change (in fact, embracing anything these days is not necessarily healthy). Nurses are taught to think critically, and it is through analytic problem solving that nurses are logically questioning policies that appear to be driven so obviously by money.

You can see that there are no easy or predictable statements to be made about the nursing job market other than that it is going through tremendous change and no one can say for certain what the results will be. But I can say this, "If you think you are ready for a challenge with change, nursing is ready for you."

ROCK AND ROLL WILL NEVER DIE—AND NEITHER WILL HOSPITAL NURSING

The Bureau of Labor Statistics (BLS) and the American Hospital Association (AHA) report in no uncertain terms that hospitals in the United States and around the world are experiencing shortages of qualified RNs. In the past it was expected that all new graduates would get their first job in a hospital. Hospitals were always the initial training ground, and they remain an excellent place to start. But new graduates today can expect to start in other settings as well. A recent nursing graduate got her first job in a home health agency working with what is called the First Steps Program. She coordinates care for pregnant women and young children. She was lucky to get the job because they don't usually hire new graduates. But because she persevered and had past volunteer experiences, she was able to get the job.

HAVE I GOT A DEAL FOR YOU: THE JOB MARKET

You might be wondering where you will work when you get out of nursing school. Of the 56.2% of nurses now working in hospitals, most work in medical-surgical units, followed by intensive care, operating rooms, and Emergency Departments. Nurses working outside hospitals work in community and public health; doctor, nurse, or group clinics; nursing homes; or roles such as nurse practitioner.

The geographic distribution of nurses is reflected in regional variations of populations and the types of health care services they need. The following list will give you an idea of where most of the nurses are working in any one region:

- New England (New Hampshire, Vermont, Maine, Massachusetts, Connecticut, Rhode Island) has the highest concentration of RNs working in hospitals and the most working in nursing homes.
- Mid-Atlantic (New Jersey, New York, Pennsylvania) has the largest portion of nurses working in student health. This area, along with the Eastern North Central states, has the second largest number of working RNs.
- Eastern South Central (Alabama, Kentucky, Mississippi, Tennessee) has the most nurses employed in community and public health. They also have more nurses under age 29 and more African-American nurses than any other region.
- Mountain (Arizona, Colorado, Idaho, Montana, Nevada, New Mexico, Utah, Wyoming) has the fewest number of working RNs but the largest portion of American Indian/Alaskan Native RNs.
- Pacific (Alaska, Hawaii, California, Oregon, Washington) has the oldest RNs (ages 50 to 64) and the most RNs from non-Caucasian backgrounds, especially Asian-Americans and Pacific Islanders.

Salaries vary by region, with nurses working in the Pacific earning the most and those in East South Central the least. Don't forget when looking at salaries to consider the cost of living. A $50,000 salary in Red Lodge, Montana, is worth a lot more than it is in New York City.

Several career guides, including the *Occupational Outlook Handbook*, expect employment opportunities for nurses to increase faster than the average for all other occupations. Nursing is expected to have the largest increase in numbers employed, and the U.S. Department of Labor expects this growth to continue. And, as we saw earlier, the need for nurses with advanced graduate training is expected to rise rapidly as well. Job vacancies occur in all settings such as in inner cities and rural locations and in the specialty areas of geriatrics, critical care, obstetrics, and surgical care. The greatest growth is expected to occur in home health and nursing homes, although it may not be as great as some anticipate; and outpatient centers are increasing as fewer procedures require an overnight stay in the hospital.

Overall you can see that the employment outlook is excellent if you choose to become a nurse. My advice is that you do some research in the region in which you want to work and check out your prospects. Keep in mind that as a nurse there are also many opportunities for travel. If you decide you want to leave the nest, there are plenty of places to land a job. Traveling nursing is an excellent choice if you want to see the world, and there are several large agencies. For example, Cross Country TravCorps will hire you after you've gotten some experience. I know two nurses who worked in international jobs earning tax-free salaries and free flights during their vacations; a nurse in Kenya who helped manage a hospital and a clinic; a nurse who chose to work night shifts in Hawaii so she could sleep on the beach during the day; and a nurse who worked a month in Kentucky, a month in New York City, a month in Los Angeles, and then returned home to Denver for a vacation before taking off again. Nurse practitioner Beth, accompanied by her husband and two school-age children, spent a year living in a remote area of Nepal, where she ran the health clinic. Beth and her family considered this experience invaluable and when they returned to the U.S., they immediately began making plans to work in Mongolia for the Peace Corps.

HOW LONG WILL IT TAKE TO GET MY FIRST JOB?

The majority of new nurses will have a job immediately on graduating from school. At Washington State University College of Nursing, nursing students had an average of two job offers at graduation and many had five or more.

IT'S NO MYSTERY: FINDING A JOB

The least likely ways to find a job are through classified advertising, on-site recruitment, or a faculty member's recommendation. The NLN claims that most new nurses find their first jobs in one of the following three ways:

1. Through prior association with an institution
2. Through their clinical site in an institution during nursing school
3. Via word of mouth

Prior Association with an Institution

Many new graduates, especially those for whom nursing is a second career, previously worked for the institution that eventually employs them as an RN. For instance, if you worked in a hospital as an x-ray technician and decided to go into nursing, it is likely that the same hospital will employ you as a new RN graduate.

This also holds true if you return to school for a graduate degree and are looking for your first job as an advanced practice nurse (APN). Nancy worked in a large hospital for many years before deciding to get her master's degree in nursing. For her graduate school research project, she developed and implemented a classification system for that hospital's cardiac care unit to help improve and speed up patient recovery and discharge. The hospital administration was so pleased with Nancy's work that they hired her back as a consultant. Encouraged, Nancy started her own business as an organizational nurse consultant. She controls her own hours, makes a good living, and loves her work.

Clinical Site During Nursing School

When you go to nursing school, you'll spend a number of weeks each term learning clinical skills. These "clinicals" take place in many different locations. If you have a clinical in the hospital, you may be in pediatrics or obstetrics or on a medical-surgical unit. If your clinical is in the community, you may be at a Public Health Department, the Visiting Nurses Association, or the public schools or in a clinic for low-income women and children. At any of your clinical sites you interact and work closely with other nurses and managers employed there. It is not uncommon for a student who does well in a clinical experience to return to the site for employment.

One student I knew in Spokane wanted more than anything to be a labor and delivery nurse when she graduated. This is an area that is very popular. This student did two clinical rotations, one in labor and delivery and one in postpartum care. She worked very hard and made an effort to get to know the other nurses. After her first year in nursing school she met with the manager of the unit and asked for a summer job as a nursing technician (a title sometimes used for nursing students; other students get a certification as a nursing aide). The manager was reluctant to hire her because she already had many requests from other students. So the student had two of her instructors, one who worked part-time in the unit, call the manager and recommend her.

She didn't get hired, but she was referred to pediatrics, where she did get the summer job. When she graduated from school, the obstetrics manager, impressed with her work in pediatrics, hired her for a part-time position on the night shift. This story is a great example of how persistence and hard work in your clinical experiences can help you find a job.

Word of Mouth

I found every job I've ever had by word of mouth. First of all, it helps to talk to a lot of people. The more people you know, the better this method works. How do you get to know nurses? Talk to the nurses at your clinical sites; go to conferences; join professional organizations and associations; volunteer for committees and community services such as blood drives, free blood pressure screenings, and aid stations at triathlons, marathons, fun runs, and other community events. To find out about professional events, call your district, state, or specialty nurses association or your local nursing school.

Read the paper to get a feel for where the jobs are located and what kind of requirements they have. For example, some jobs require certain certifications. Some of these, such as advanced cardiac life support (ACLS) or cardiopulmonary resuscitation (CPR) instructor, can be earned before you are an experienced nurse. Once you've discovered where the jobs are or what you would like to do, start working toward that goal by getting to know people and keeping your eyes and ears open for opportunities.

I am a firm believer in this method because most nurses I know got their first job not by applying to a personnel office, but by talking to other nurses, especially the nurse managers. They decided where they wanted to work, called the nurse manager, and set up an appointment to talk. You can arrange these meetings while still in school to gather information about what managers are looking for in an employee. Following are some good questions to ask:

- What does it take to be an RN in that area?
- Are there things you can be doing to prepare for a job there?
- Do they hire nursing students during the summers?
- Do they hire new graduates?

This is an effective way to develop relationships and to stay in contact with the people who have the most power to influence your eventual employment.

GI JANES OR JOES: THE MILITARY

From the Crusades of the Middle Ages to Florence Nightingale making history in the Crimea, to the Korean War and the Vietnam conflict, nurses have been a vital part of the military. The Red Cross, first established in Italy and inspired by Nightingale, was later started in the United States by nurse Clara Barton. It was the source of over 2000 military nurses who served in the Civil War (including author Louisa May Alcott). In 1901 the government formed the Army Nurse Corps to meet the military's growing need for nurses.

To this day the military trains and employs nurses in peacetime and in war. If you are interested in serving in the military, I strongly urge you to explore this option. The military can help you with school expenses and employ you as an officer after you graduate. There is ample opportunity to advance in rank and have your tuition to graduate school paid for as well.

I never considered this option because I never regarded myself as the military type. Perhaps I never gave it a fair chance, but the time commitment, military training, and tightly structured order did not appeal to me. That is not at all to say the military would not work for you, however. I know several very bright nursing students who applied and were accepted by the Army or Navy. It was a good opportunity for them financially and professionally. One student, Joanne, served in the military after graduation from nursing school. She worked in medical tents in the desert in Afghanistan. Her experiences have inspired several other students to go into military nursing. For further information, contact your local recruiter or write for information.

NURSE'S CAPS: GONE WITH THE WIND

Nurses don't wear caps anymore; but they do wear many hats in terms of the roles they take on. At one time, nursing was limited to hospitals, public health clinics, and war zones. Today nurses work in these places and many more. After graduating from nursing school, you will probably choose a specialty area such as community health, home health, obstetrics, emergency, geriatrics, medical-surgical, occupational health, operating room, pediatrics, psychiatric, or rehabilitation. These are examples of the diversity of nursing hats you can choose to wear, but, within any one of these areas nurses also wear many different hats.

For example, as a critical care nurse in an intensive care unit (ICU) you might take care of patients; work on a committee to develop discharge criteria; manage a nurse's aide; instruct a newly employed RN; teach your patient's family about their loved one's illness; provide grief counseling; or coordinate care with doctors (most critical care patients have several doctors at any one time), pharmacists, and social workers. In addition, you may be assigned the job of making the work schedule for the upcoming holiday season. After work you attend a meeting of your professional organization that includes an update on a clinical topic of interest. The next morning you may attend a board meeting of your local women and children's shelter and write a letter to your congressional representative to support legislation protecting patient safety.

It's a busy life and it isn't lived only in the hospital ICU. Nurses do many things in many settings. Picture yourself working internationally with refugees and immigrants, providing relief work in famine areas, or giving vaccinations and assisting in eye surgery for orphans in Romania. One of the biggest advantages to being a nurse is the number of opportunities available. I recently attended a nursing conference where the keynote speaker, Marie Manthey, advised, "Don't go into nursing for money, power, or prestige, but for the value of helping—one human being to another." The beauty of nursing is that there are so many ways to do this, and I can't think of any other career that offers the same flexibility and rewards.

IN AND OUT: WHAT'S NEW?

Health care is as rich in new opportunities as the old system was in jobs. New technologies have created a wealth of new nursing specialties such as computer information systems and genetics. Changing health care systems are greatly increasing the need for nurse practitioners, who provide primary care, and case managers, who coordinate the care for patients with complex chronic conditions. Because of health care changes, nurses are also needed to evaluate and make public policy in regard to the development of new systems. The number of people, especially children, with no health care coverage is increasing; and nurses are needed to help remedy this growing problem. In short, the new opportunities for nurses are in the areas of technology, health care delivery systems, and policy analysis and politics.

Technology
Genetics

With the advent of the Human Genome Project (an international attempt to map the entire human genome) and the continuously improving technology used to identify genes responsible for disease, the entire field of genetics is booming. Understanding basic genetic principles is a shortfall for many nurses, so this topic is an area of specialization that you could choose. Nurses also provide genetic counseling and teaching to patients, work with children and adults with genetic diseases, and do research in genetics. There is a need for well-versed nurse ethicists because many problems involving privacy and decision-making are accompanying these new genetic discoveries. The International Society of Nurses in Genetics, a small specialty group, encourages nurses to keep up with the changes because they have an impact on nursing practice.

For example, privacy becomes an issue if genetic screening eventually allows us to predetermine whether a person is at risk for certain conditions such as heart disease. Who has a right to know about this? Employers? Insurance companies? Other family members? It's possible that health care insurers would refuse coverage if they knew that a person were likely to develop a costly disease; employers might be reluctant to hire a person if they thought that a genetic condition could cause excess sick time; and biologic family members may or may not want to know what their outlook is for being at risk for receiving or carrying a genetic defect. Decisions about what to do with genetic information raise many legal and ethical questions.

Another example of technologic change is birth defect screening. Although some screening is already done routinely, the potential for more is occurring as geneticists rapidly discover gene locations for diseases such as spina bifida, cystic fibrosis, and Huntington's disease. Difficult questions arise, such as should prospective parents be told, and, if they are told, should they be advised on abortion as an option? Routine gender identification is another issue with ethical implications. If it were easy to determine the gender of the unborn child, might parents opt for abortion to control whether they have a boy or a girl?

In the mid-1990s the American Nurses Association (ANA) Center for Ethics and Human Rights conducted research on the management of genetic information and published a booklet called *Managing Genetic Information: Policies for U.S. Nurses*. The booklet covers the importance of understanding genetics, guidelines for dealing with genetic information, and privacy issues. The ANA currently works with the American Medical Association and the National Human Genome Research Institute to provide genetic education to all health care professionals.

Information Sciences (Informatics)

It is no news to anyone that we are living in the information age. We are surrounded by an abundant and overwhelming amount of information coming from places such as the Internet, but it is largely disorganized. Thus there are numerous opportunities for nurses not only to organize information but in to make it accessible, meaningful, and relevant to the user. Designing computer systems requires advanced computer skills and knowledge of nursing and health care. Nurses interested in technical fields should take elective, or graduate, courses in computer and information science. You can also get a Masters in Nursing with Informatics as your specialty.

Transplant Nurse

Transplant nurses work in the area of organ transplantation. They coordinate and provide care before, during, and after surgery. Nurses do a great deal of teaching with patients, families, and in the community. Following is an example of a job posting from the website of the International Transplant Nurses Society (www.itns.org/):

Kidney and Pancreas Transplant Coordinators

Posted April 25, 2006

University of Minnesota Medical Center, Fairview in Minneapolis is a progressive leader providing the best in innovative care. We have a rewarding opportunity for a self-motivated Kidney and Pancreas Transplant Coordinator. In this role, you will serve as the primary care coordinator for patients in the post-transplant phase of care management, as well as serve as a liaison with transplant physicians. Qualified applicants must possess an RN license, BSN, and 3-5 years of recent critical care or transplant experience. This position requires a highly motivated individual who demonstrates excellent leadership, communication, and organizational skills. If you are looking for career advancement and the opportunity to be a valued member of a multi-disciplinary team, this is the job for you!

Health Care Delivery Systems

Advanced Practice Nurses

APNs (nurse practitioners, nurse midwives, clinical nurse specialists, and nurse anesthetists) are not new, but certain areas of their practice are. APNs are becoming key players in the changing health care environment, especially when the emphasis is on saving money. One way to save money is to keep people from getting sick and, when they do get sick, to keep them from getting sicker. For example, studies have shown that nurse practitioners reduce the number of patients that need to be hospitalized by providing extensive illness prevention education. Insurance companies also report an increasing demand by the public for these nurse providers.

Entrepreneur

It is becoming more and more common to find nurses who are going out and doing it on their own (that is, becoming entrepreneurs or small business owners). Some have developed patient care products such as a better fastener to secure endotracheal tubes; others hire themselves out as consultants (a nurse who delivers lactation consultation for new mothers is one example, and a nurse who collects and analyzes data on the effectiveness of a certain procedure in a doctor's office is another); and still others set up their own clinic, counseling center, or health spa.

Manager of Care

Nurses are in the perfect position to be managers of health services. They understand the needs of patients, and they have vast experience working with many other members of the health care team. Essentially nurses work as managers and coordinators of care, no matter what type of job they have. To help save health care dollars, a growing interest in streamlining care through good management has arisen. Nurses who work in case management coordinate the care of a patient from hospitalization to home. They ensure that patients are educated and have what they need to get well; they also ensure that services are not duplicated (a big, costly problem in the past). Other nurses manage care for populations or groups of people. For instance, overseeing the day-to-day health of people with chronic conditions such as heart failure, diabetes, or asthma has been shown to be extremely cost-effective. In this capacity you can work for a health care management organization, the public health services, a clinic, a hospital, or a home health agency.

Policy and Politics
Policy Analyst

Health care systems need people to find solutions to numerous problems that arise in health care. Nurses, whose focus is on health and wellness and who put policy into action every day in their practice, have a great deal to contribute to health care policymaking. Most large health care organizations, government agencies, and private insurance companies employ policy analysts. If you have a bent toward political science or problem analysis, you may find a niche here.

Cultural Diversity and Cultural Competency

With increasing diversity in the U.S., there is tremendous need for nurses who are culturally sensitive and competent concerning diverse populations. An experienced nurse who is bilingual will always have a job, and one who can teach others about cultural diversity is a close runner-up. All health care professionals are trying to improve themselves and their organizations in this area, and as a nurse with a holistic perspective, you will be in a good position to provide these services.

Other new roles are also appearing with changes in science, technology, and society. When I went to nursing school, we never discussed special health needs of the gay, lesbian, bisexual, transgendered (GLBT) community. Today these needs are part of the nursing curriculum. Working with vulnerable populations (that is, those underserved or underrepresented), is a growing area in nursing. Specialty areas of practice are being created. Other examples include end-of-life care; homelessness; domestic violence; and alternative health, such as acupuncture, healing touch, and complementary medicines.

Legal Nursing

Legal nursing is a booming field. Wendy is a nurse who has worked in community health, including long-term care. She owned and ran a long-term care facility for many years. She eventually grew tired of this work and took some courses to become a specialist in legal nursing. She is self-employed and hired as a consultant by lawyers to be an expert witness in health care lawsuit cases. She likes being independent, and she makes approximately $100.00 per hour (this could be much more, depending on the area in which you worked). Her qualifications for the job are as follows:

1. She is an RN and therefore an expert in health care.
2. She has extensive nursing experience at different levels in the community.

3. She has worked in nursing education.
4. She is certified as a Life Care Planner, a Rehabilitation RN, and a Case Manager.

The thing she doesn't like about this work is that the plaintiff's lawyers are always trying to discredit her. They look for inconsistencies in her work; thus she has to be meticulous in her preparation. She also travels a lot, and that keeps her away from home more than she would like. Wendy loves her work and says that she thinks this is a growing field in nursing. She doesn't have the time to take many of the cases that she's offered. She has more work than she can, or wants, to do.

Forensic Nursing

Another popular and growing area in health care and nursing is forensics, although it is probably not like you see it on TV. Forensic nurses have an advanced degree or a master's degree in nursing with a focus on forensics. Forensic nursing works with the health care system and legal systems. A forensic nurse might work with children who are victims of abuse, women who are victims of domestic violence or rape, and inmates in a prison. Just about any criminal case that involves health (for example, food and drug tampering and traumatic injuries) is the jurisdiction of a forensics nurse. Investigating crime is a major focus. For example, a nurse working with abused children will investigate the crime and manage a child's care through hospitalization and foster care. The nurse will often work with the children again in court when testifying about the case.

To be a forensic nurse you need special education, a willingness and ability to work collaboratively with other professionals and with extremes in human behavior, and a psychiatric nursing background.

International Health

Working internationally is also a growing area of nursing. There is a nursing shortage globally, and it is worsening in many places as nurses are recruited to fill the needs in countries such as the United States and Great Britain. In Africa this is becoming a real problem as Africans have many health care needs exacerbated by the HIV/AIDS epidemic. Issues being worked on by nurses internationally include:

- Nutrition and older people
- Birth registration
- Childhood nutrition
- The girl child
- Maternal and infant nutrition
- Prevention of child abuse
- Safeguarding the childhood of children
- Displaced persons (refugees)
- Gender and health (including men's health)
- Health and human rights
- The health of indigenous peoples
- Immunization safety
- International trade (this includes affects of International trade agreements and trade-related aspects of intellectual property rights)
- Mental health

- Poverty and health
- Safe household water

NURSE MIGRATION TRENDS

Migration is a problem in the nursing profession because of the nursing shortage, but it is quite understandable from the individual nurse's viewpoint. Nurses tend to leave their homes for jobs overseas when they live in rural, low-income areas. They tend to move from developing to industrialized countries (for example, a nurse who moves from Tanzania to England). Industrialized countries such as the United States and England recruit nurses from developing countries to meet their shortage.

According to the International Council of Nurses, nurses migrate to find:
1. Improved learning and practice opportunities.
2. Better quality of life, pay and working conditions.
3. Personal safety.

The advantages and disadvantages of this trend are outlined in Box 9-1.

Many of the new and growing opportunities for nurses are related to changes in technology, the nursing shortage, and social and political changes. Change is often accompanied by ethical dilemmas. The nurse migration issue is such an ethical dilemma. One way to look at richer countries recruiting nurses from poorer countries is that they are taking advantage of poorer countries. But, on the other hand, individual nurses in the poorer countries have a right to improve their lives, even if it means possible worsening of health care in their own countries. This is a dilemma. Chapter 10 will discuss ethics in greater detail.

BOX 9-1	International Nurse Migration: Advantages and Disadvantages

PROS	CONS
Educational and professional opportunities	Brain and/or skills drain away from the country of origin
Personal and occupational safety	Closure of health facilities due to nursing shortages in a given area
Better working conditions	Overworked nurses left practicing in depleted areas
Improved quality of life	Potentially abusive recruitment and employment practices
Transcultural nursing workforce (e.g., racial and ethnic diversity) for new country	Vulnerable status of migrants in new countries
Cultural sensitivity and competence in care	Loss of national economic investment in human resource development
Stimulation of nurse-friendly recruitment and contract conditions	
Personal development	
Global economic development	
Improved knowledge base and brain "gain"	
Sustained maintenance and development of family members in the country of origin	

From International Council of Nurses (ICN): *Career moves and migration: critical questions*. Geneva, Switzerland, 2002, ICN. Retrieved June 21, 2006, from www.icn.ch/CareerMovesMigangl.pdf.

Chapter

10

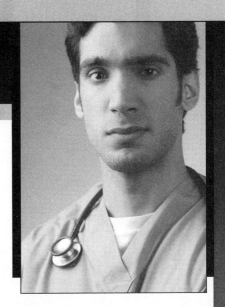

Working for a Living

Some of the issues you will face as a working nurse are included in this chapter. To give you a clear picture, I've included what registered nurses (RNs) around the country are saying about being a nurse in the current political and economic climate.

WHAT NURSES SAY ABOUT NURSING

The American Nurses Association (ANA) Staffing Survey polled 7300 nurses in 2001. The responses were voluntary, so the results do not represent the views of all, or even a majority, of nurses; but they do provide an idea of what some nurses around the country are experiencing. Following are some of the findings:

- Approximately 56% of nurses thought time for patient care had decreased.
- A majority of respondents said that increased patient loads or the number of patients they had to care for caused a decrease in the quality of care.
- Approximately 75% of nurses thought that the quality of nursing care had decreased in the past 2 years. Approximately 11.5% thought it had improved.
- The top three things that were causing quality of care to decrease were: (1) inadequate staffing, (2) decreased nurse work satisfaction, and (3) delays in providing care.
- When asked what nurses had experienced in the past 2 years, the answers most frequently cited were skipping meals and breaks in order to care for patients, feeling an increased pressure to accomplish work, working overtime, and stress-related illness.
- Many nurses said they would not recommend nursing as a career.

It is important to realize that, although these survey results are not positive, they do indicate that people are paying attention to the problem. Also realize that approximately 48% of respondents worked in an acute care hospital setting. Only approximately 4% were researchers, educators, or advanced practice nurses. Further, approximately 23% had been nurses for 25 years or longer. Only approximately 9.7% were younger than 30 years old.

The American Nurse Credentialing Center, the leading nursing credentialing organization in the United States, published 2004 survey results from 1000 nurses responding to questions about their opinions of their workplace environment. The greatest number of nurses, approximately 83%, felt largely negative about their workplace. Another approximately 12% had positive feelings, and approximately 8% were neutral. The top issues that respondents said affected their opinions were quality of patient care, quality of nursing leaders, and human resources (personnel) policies and programs.

Karen is an example of this. She is the nurse manager of an oncology unit, and she told me she was thinking of leaving nursing and opening a flower shop. When I asked why, she said she didn't like being a manager and missed patient care. I asked her why she didn't just go back to being a staff nurse and she said, "Because with the changes in staffing on the unit, I couldn't care for patients anymore the way it should be done. With the addition of aides, the RNs have so many more patients to oversee that there isn't time to take good care of them. I wouldn't have a real handle on each person's care." It is a tragedy that expert nurses like Karen are thinking of leaving nursing. I wish all nurses would stay and fight for what they know is the right way to provide care, but I also know that many either do not feel empowered to do so or are just too tired after a day at work.

The survey results can be discouraging, but to me they signal the need for a new direction. Nurses are the experts in patient care, and if they think that care is compromised, they must take action to find a remedy. In the long run, not only will the remedy improve patient care, but the care will be more efficient. Administrators who are responsible for staffing decisions must listen carefully to what nurses say and what their research is beginning to reveal.

The health care system is becoming more complex, and with it more complex jobs are evolving. Nurses with training in research, advanced sciences, and communication will have the best opportunities for career mobility.

LET'S MAKE A DEAL:
COLLECTIVE BARGAINING AND CONTRACTS

I hope the title of this section doesn't turn you off, because these three words, "collective bargaining contract," are vital to nursing, and you should be prepared to work under a negotiated contract. Your state nurses association through the United American Nurses and the AFL/CIO is often the bargaining agent for nurse's contracts, although sometimes nurses vote to have a traditional labor union negotiate for them instead. Workplaces have two kinds of membership: mandatory and optional. In a mandatory membership you belong to the bargaining unit as a condition of employment (called a closed shop); in an optional setup membership is a choice, but, whether you are a member or not, you are covered by the contract.

At the hospital where I worked for 10 years, over 65% of the nurses were optional members of the nurses association. Our contract covered everything from salary, benefits, and use of sick time to layoff procedures. The 35% who were not members received the same terms under the contract. It is easy to understand how the paying members resented those who didn't pay dues but who received the same benefits. Nevertheless, labor laws allow this; at every contract negotiation we tried to get a closed shop, but the administration would not agree. So we diligently worked year-round to convince nonmembers to become members.

The purpose of collective bargaining is not only to negotiate equitable salaries and safe working conditions but also to protect patients. It allows nurses, who are the patient care experts, to have a voice in how things are done.

One reason nurses may be dissatisfied with their workplace is the risk for injuries. An unsafe workplace for nurses will contribute to poorer quality patient care. RNs are at the highest risk of any other person in the workplace for back injuries—higher even than construction workers. The benefit of having a negotiated contract is that it puts into writing the conditions agreed on by nurses and administrators. Everyone is held accountable. Following are examples of real contract wording excerpted from the website of the organization United American Nurses (UAN), AFL-CIO (www.uannurse.org/highlights/health.html):

- UAN RNs at Samaritan Medical Center have contract language guaranteeing that "the employer shall provide adequate numbers and availability of [patient] lifting devices" to prevent back injuries.
- Nurses at Fairview Hospitals in Minnesota ratified language requiring the hospitals to prevent violence and verbal abuse through patient risk assessments, an annual course on de-escalation, behavior management, physical protection, and a trained response team.
- Staff nurses have contract language banning the use of Cidex (glutaraldehyde), a widely used disinfectant that can cause asthma, rashes, nausea, and headaches.
- Every nurse at Children's Hospitals and Clinics in St. Paul is "allowed to decide if fatigue prevents her/him from delivering safe patient care."

Over 10 years ago, journalist Suzanne Gordon, during a 1996 interview about her book, *Life Support: Three Nurses on the Front Lines* (1997, Little, Brown), encouraged nurses, "We have spent a century articulating and developing the science and art of nursing and will not give this up." Gordon recommends that nurses work together (through state and national associations) to uphold their high standards for quality patient care.

Essential to working with or without a contract is the principle that all involved, administrators and nurses alike, have a common goal—excellent patient care. The Washington State Nurses Association and Sacred Heart Medical Center prefaced their contract with the following statement:

> The main purpose of this Agreement is to set forth the understanding reached between parties in establishing equitable employment standards and an orderly system of employer-employee relationships.

Good communication is critical to maintaining a working relationship that fosters and supports the services you and your employer are providing. Contracts can protect you and your patients, but if you work without one, take extra care to be familiar with your Nursing Practice Act and state employment regulations.

WHY SHOULD YOU JOIN THE AMERICAN NURSES ASSOCIATION? THE DYNAMIC DUO: POWER AND POLITICS

Even though many nurses do not go into nursing with the idea that they will be politically active, most want to have control over their practice. If nurses do not have this control, then others tell us how to do our work. What is needed is a good deal of education, knowledge, and research about nursing, together with a unified voice to fully control our practice. Nothing can replace research-based information and group action in creating strong support for nursing. Data presented to the public and to Congress will help RNs gain professional power and political clout. In this way nurses can work in the political arena to influence and write laws and in their own workplaces to protect their patients and practice nursing as only nurses know best how to do.

The ANA represents RNs in the United States. The following mission statement, which is excerpted from the organization's website (www.nursingworld.org), explains its main goals of helping nurses and patients:

> The mission of the American Nurses Association is to work for the improvement of health standards and availability of health care services for all people, foster high standards for nursing, stimulate and promote the professional development of nurses, and advance their economic and general welfare.

Membership is obtained by paying annual dues that are regulated by each state association. In the state of Washington, dues vary, depending on employment status such as whether you work part-time, full-time, are retired; or if the ANA affiliate United American Nurses AFL/CIO negotiates your employment contract (the ANA also serves as a collective bargaining agent for nurses). Membership benefits also cover a subscription to the *American Nurse*. To join, call or write, and you can be put in touch with your state association; or check the website (nursingworld.org) for more information.

I often hear nurses talk about the importance of working together to make improvements in health care and in the nursing profession. The expression "united we stand, divided we fall" holds as true for nurses as for other groups. Working together, nurses are much more powerful than if they try to bring about change alone; a strong ANA leads to increased power for all nurses, whether it is improving the standards of nursing care, protecting nurses' jobs, or promoting public health through immunization campaigns, patient safety legislation, or education.

NURSES ARE PROFESSIONALS

Nursing is a profession that has its own code of conduct, its own philosophic views, and its own place in the health care team. Nurses are independent. They work under their own license and not under that of a physician. That means that nurses are completely responsible for their work. A nurse can't say that the reason she or he did something wrong was that the doctor ordered the wrong treatment or procedure. The nurse is expected to know if an order is wrong, and, if she or he doesn't understand it, to get more information. Nurses never act without full knowledge. Nurses care for individual patients but also for groups of people such as families, groups of people, communities, and even populations.

For example, when I worked in cardiac rehabilitation, I worked with individuals. But I also worked for a group of people with heart disease. I worked to prevent heart disease by promoting healthy activities such as exercise and a proper diet. I belonged to state and national groups that promote heart health such as the American Heart Association. If any legislative activity came up, I'd write to my congressional representative to ask them to support a bill. An example of this might be legislation to require schools to serve healthy diets, to take the pop machines out of the school, or to require students to get some exercise every day.

You can see that as a nurse I am responsible for much more than my individual patient. These responsibilities change with new science, the shifting priorities of our society, and political changes. Nurses are experts in health care and as such need to keep up on local and national health care issues. Can you think of any? Look at the newspaper and you will find them.

WHAT PEOPLE THINK ABOUT HEALTH CARE
AND HOW HEALTHY THEY ARE

The results of a national survey called *Consumers' Experiences With Patient Safety and Quality Information* were published in 2004. The results found that 40% of American consumers of health care services thought the quality of health care has worsened in the last 5 years, due in part to medical errors. Consumers thought that the most important issues affecting medical error rates were workload, stress, or fatigue among health professionals (74%); too little time spent with patients (70%); and too few nurses (69%). This survey was sponsored by the Kaiser Family Foundation, the Agency for Healthcare Research and Quality, and the Harvard School of Public Health.

In 2006 a study compared the health of Caucasian non-Hispanic, middle-age Americans, and British people. Despite the fact that the United States spends much more on health care than the British, Americans are less healthy. Americans are almost twice as likely to have diabetes and higher rates of hypertension, heart disease, cancer, lung disease, and strokes. Everyone connected to the study was surprised by the findings, and no one able to say why there is such a difference. This study was on the front page of most major newspapers and on major television news stations. What do Americans think about our health care system now? Do you think nurses have anything to do with this?

Groundbreaking nursing research studies are beginning to make a connection between nurses and quality of care among hospital patients. One such study, published in 2003 by Dr. Linda Aiken and colleagues from the University of Pennsylvania,[*] found that patients cared for by RNs with bachelor's degrees in nursing (BSNs) had lower death rates than those cared for by RNs with less education. Another study found that, when nurses had more than four patients to care for at any one time, the incidence of complications, including death, increased significantly.

Today and in the future being a nurse means taking on a great responsibility. Some of the health care issues that nurses are especially concerned with include the following:

- Access to health care
- Quality of health care
- Equity of health care

ETHICS—OR WHAT'S RIGHT AND WHAT'S WRONG?

Ethics is a big concern in nursing and health care. Ethics is the understanding of how decisions are made. Ethics is based on morals and values. Morals are what you believe to be right and wrong. Ethical decisions are based on what you, an organization, or a society thinks is right and wrong. Cultural perspective plays a big role in how an individual or community views morality. Within a community there can be variation as well. You only have to think about issues such as abortion and capital punishment. Should individuals be able to act on what they think, or do they have to defer to what the community thinks? This gets into the issue of individual versus community rights. When you think about it, you can see how complicated this can get.

There are many new health care technologies that add to the dilemmas. It is common for nurses to experience these dilemmas. For example, we have the ability to keep a person alive on life support for a long time. An 85-year-old who has had surgery to repair a broken hip experiences complications after surgery. The surgical site becomes infected, and the patient develops pneumonia. The patient, now on prolonged bedrest, develops a blood clot in one leg. The clot breaks free and moves to the heart and lungs. The patient does not die but is placed on a mechanical breathing device, a ventilator, with many intravenous medications to stabilize blood pressure and heart rate. Further, the patient is given antibiotics for the surgical site infection.

Without going into too many details, everything done to help the patient takes a toll. The antibiotics create other problems, as does the ventilator, the immobility of bedrest, and just being in the hospital for an extended time. It might seem easy to think about what is right regarding the patient care, but consider the reality. You are the nurse. The patient's daughter says that the patient has had a good life and life support should be terminated. She says, "He has been happy, and he told me once he didn't want to be like this. You have to stop everything right now— I insist!" The patient's wife, his second, and not the mother of the children, says, "Do everything you can for him. He would want to fight it to the end." Then the

[*]Aiken LH et al: Educational levels of hospital nurses and surgical patient mortality, JAMA 290(12): 1617-1623, 2003.

BOX **10-1**	**ICN Code of Ethics for Nurses: Preamble**

An international code of ethics for nurses was first adopted by the International Council of Nurses (ICN) in 1953. It has been revised and reaffirmed at various times since, most recently with this review and revision completed in 2005.

Nurses have four fundamental responsibilities: to promote health, to prevent illness, to restore health and to alleviate suffering. The need for nursing is universal.

Inherent in nursing is respect for human rights, including cultural rights, the right to life and choice, to dignity and to be treated with respect. Nursing care is respectful of and unrestricted by considerations of age, colour, creed, culture, disability or illness, gender, sexual orientation, nationality, politics, race or social status.

Nurses render health services to the individual, the family and the community and co-ordinate their services with those of related groups.

From International Council of Nurses (ICN): *The ICN code of ethics for nurses*, Geneva, Switzerland, 2005, ICN. Retrieved June 21, 2006, from www.icn.ch/icncode.pdf.

son says, "His wife doesn't know him like we do; he would never want this. You should try the treatments for 1 more week." Everyone is arguing. You wonder if the patient had a living will.

What do you do? The doctor is very busy and has talked to the individual members of the family but not to all of them at once. The patient's condition is worsening. What is the right thing to do, and who gets to decide what "right" means? That's ethics. It is not easy, and it is not black and white. You may have your personal views about right and wrong, and the right decision might be very clear to you, but as a nurse you cannot use your views to judge others.

To learn more about ethics and nursing, review the ANA *Code of Ethics for Nurses With Interpretive Statements* revised in 2001 (www.nursingworld.org/ethics/ecode.htm). Another example of nursing ethics is provided by the International Council of Nurses (ICN). The ICN is the global professional nursing organization. Box 10-1 contains the preamble to the ICN Code of Ethics. It will give you an idea of nursing on an international level. Consider whether you agree with these codes. Do your values coincide with these codes? Reading the codes will also give you another way to look at nursing and to understand what nursing is all about.

Chapter

11

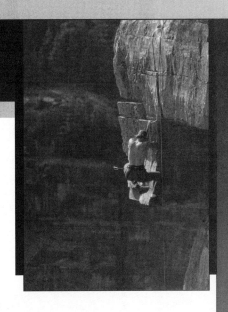

Survival in the Workplace

At this point you may be thinking that being a nurse is not easy in a sometimes unrecognized and under-rewarded profession. You are right. It requires a challenging education, hard work, dedication, and a willingness to be politically astute, if not politically active.

You are also right if you're thinking that nursing is diverse, rewarding, and well-paying and offers flexible hours and the opportunity to work just about any place on the globe that you can imagine. Finally, nursing serves the public good. If you choose, you can greatly benefit the many who are underserved and need good nurses: minorities, women, children, elderly; and those who live in poverty or are war torn or disenfranchised.

STAYING ALIVE

While you are doing these great things, there is one basic requirement, or prescription, that you must follow—you must take care of yourself. You must have your needs (for example, nurturing your feelings of self-worth, caring for your spirit, and promoting a healthy body) met outside the work environment. Any nurse you talk to will tell you that, if you do not take care of yourself, you cannot take care of others; although many nurses, doctors, physical therapists, and other health care professionals do not follow this golden rule. But ask yourself, "How can I take care of others and teach them to care for themselves if I don't know how to take care of myself?"

I think of it as the "care equation." If you leave yourself out of the formula, the results (quality patient care) will not be accurate. I learned this rule the hard way. When I first worked in critical care, I was fascinated with the machines, the monitors, and all the exciting technical skills. I loved talking to the patients and the families, but it was the ability to work in emergencies using all the equipment and medications that interested me the most; that was the ultimate challenge and thrill. For instance, each shift one nurse from our cardiac intensive care unit was designated to function as the house code nurse. When any other unit in the hospital had a code, that nurse would go and be in charge of cardiopulmonary resuscitation, medications, defibrillation, and anything else that had to be done.

It's no exaggeration to say that I lived for the day when I could be code nurse. It took me 2 years, but I felt at the top of my profession when I could go to another unit and use my expertise to direct others. So what happened? Over the next 7 years I accomplished all this and much more, when suddenly, or so it seemed, I started feeling depressed. I would go home from work with a lump in my throat and drive to work with butterflies in my stomach. It became so stressful that I had to take a 3-month leave of absence, during which I spent most of the time allowing myself to feel all the sadness that had built up over the years and years of seeing tragedy after tragedy and dealing with conflicts with doctors and administrators (mostly doctors). I also rested from all the overtime I did to help in short staffing situations and to make extra money.

I had "burnout," a term with which I'm sure you're familiar. It is used in different ways, but here it refers to the feelings of a nurse who cannot care for others anymore without harming herself or himself because she or he has become psychologically, emotionally, or physically run-down. It occurs in many different situations and to many different kinds of people.

What I learned from this was, simply, that taking care of yourself is essential to taking care of others. For me this meant working in an area outside of critical care. I moved to cardiac rehabilitation, where I spent a great deal of time teaching patients and families about heart disease and thinking how good it felt not to be in constant life-or-death situations. However, there are many other nurses who thrive in the critical care or emergency environment while being able to take good care of themselves. So the important thing is to discover what works best for you by staying attuned to your thoughts and feelings, eating a healthy diet and exercising, and talking with other nurses or friends. As a nurse you are closely involved with people in all phases of trauma and loss. It is not at all uncommon for nurses to be rescuers or just plain super-nurses. After all, it feels good to help people, it's very satisfying, and it can make you feel good about yourself. Certainly there is much joy in nursing; I do not mean to negate that. In fact, the job I have now is wonderful—even fun—most of the time, despite the sadness of disease and occasionally death.

There are few other professions that offer the same freedom to do the intelligent, meaningful work that nursing does (that is, and still earn a living). Unfortunately, there are some working conditions that are not supportive of nurses and that may precipitate burnout. If you learn to become aware of your feelings and how to deal with the stresses as they come along, you will be better prepared. If you are not aware of any specific stress, look for the following indicators that often signal emotional overload: not sleeping well, changes in your eating habits, feeling tired all the time, frequent irritability or sadness, and feelings of anxiety. Anytime you are overwhelmed by your feelings, you should get help by talking to a friend, parent, or counselor (many of whom are nurses). Caring for yourself needs to be practiced, and the perfect place to start is when you're in nursing school!

IS ANYTHING ALL RIGHT OR ALL WRONG?

If you tend to go through life thinking about things only in terms of black and white or right and wrong, being a nurse is sure to change your mind. You will discover more shades of gray than you ever thought possible. Imagine taking care of someone who has an incurable disease, has had multiple surgeries resulting in a stroke, and is unable to speak or move. The cost in sheer dollars alone of caring for this person in a hospital, in an extended-care facility, or even at home is extreme. But what about quality of life? One family member may tell you, "She wanted to go peacefully; she didn't want all the machines, tubes, or life support. Just let her go." Another family member says, "You've got to do everything possible; she wanted to live. Besides, it's not right to just pull the plug." You have taken care of this patient on and off for weeks and know the suffering of both the patient and the family. The doctors have said there is little or no chance of recovery, yet they insist on continuing to try high-tech treatments. What do you do? Is there a right way to proceed? Would the fact that the patient is 95 years old affect your thinking? What if she were 5 years old or an infant? Who should get to decide and why?

Nursing is full of these situations, and they have led to a growing specialty in health care called ethics. Chapter 9 discussed problems connected to the growing field of ethics in genetics, but ethical concerns crop up in all areas of health care, including providing health care, how organizations are managed, how you treat your co-workers, and how they treat you. Essentially ethical concerns are an inescapable part of a nurse's job. You will study health care ethics in nursing school because it is important to be clear, or as clear as you can be, about your personal values and morals, and to realize that they will change with time and experience. Educating yourself on the philosophies and methods for dealing with a variety of people and situations will help you be sensitive to others' needs as well as to your own.

DIFFICULT PEOPLE: PATIENTS AND CO-WORKERS

Nurses deal with difficult people; they may be co-workers, patients, or a patient's family and friends.

Usually difficult people merely think or act differently than you do or in ways that really annoy you. In nursing you will cross paths with a great number of people, and there will always be those who bother you to different degrees. Some are minor pains, whereas others are gigantic canker sores cracking and bleeding every time you go near them. I like the way I heard a Buddhist monk explain it: people just throw the knives at you, but you must be the one to pick them up and stab yourself. In other words, examine your own motives and reactions before you label a person difficult. Generally, though, if you feel bad when you interact with someone time after time, and if a personality conflict is not the cause, the person may have problems that cause them to interact with others poorly.

I've had doctors hang up the phone on me in the middle of the night; I've had managers angry at me for not doing something the way they wanted it done; I've had patients say things to me that made the hair on the back of my neck stand up; I've seen family members come in to visit patients drunk or on drugs; and I've caught patients lighting up cigarettes with their oxygen on (a very dangerous fire hazard). One important step in coping with situations like these is to learn to recognize your biases, to get help from a co-worker if you need to talk, and, if that doesn't help, to talk to your manager, continuing on up the ladder of your organization until you get results. Don't forget to always document the problem as objectively as possible. The same applies to nursing school. You have rights—even though you are a nursing student. Go to the website for the National Student Nurses Association to get a copy of its *Student's Bill of Rights* (www.nsna.org/pubs/billofrights.asp); a copy of this document is printed on the inside front cover of this book.

More dangerous is the possibility of physical abuse from patients or co-workers. Safety in the workplace is an issue that is gaining national attention from all nursing organizations. The number of assaults and work-related injuries is on the rise. You should no more accept abusive language or action from a patient than from a physician or other co-worker. Do not let abusive behavior be dismissed, even if it means going above your immediate supervisor's head. In the end, your workplace is responsible for your safety.

The nurse can still also encounter sexual abuse or harassment. I wish the whole issue had been clearer in my early nursing days. I can't tell you the number of times various doctors and even men who were nurses made offensive comments or gave me a quick peck on the cheek. It makes my blood boil just to think of it and how helpless I felt. I kept thinking, "Oh well, this is just part of the job; nothing I can do about it." Luckily those days are over. Become familiar with the laws on sexual harassment and employer policies; fear not, they are stringent enough to motivate any employer to take your complaints seriously.

CHANGE DIRECTION, OR YOU'LL END UP WHERE YOU ARE HEADED

This old Chinese proverb is easily applied to nursing because one advantage in being a nurse is that you can change directions without ever leaving your career. You never need to feel stuck because there are always job alternatives unless you live in a completely isolated place where there is only one nursing job, you have it, and there is no way you can move. But even in that situation, today there may be hope: the Internet. You can start your own website, create a home page of nursing advice, publish articles and information, and advertise to sell them. It is being done by others; why not you? If you hate to write, try developing a telephone counseling business, or better yet, find an unmet need in your community and develop a new nursing service.

Few of the nurses I know are doing the same thing they did, or thought they would do, when they were in nursing school. Be brave and branch out, and don't ever think it is too late for you. Many of the nurses I know who recently graduated with their master's degrees are 50 years or older. After all, that's the age of the baby boomers. America is aging, and as it does, seniors are more healthy, active, and youthful than ever. Elders are downhill-skiing and snowboarding, riding elephants in India, and biking through Nepal, so why not nursing school and a career change? Why not graduate school and an advanced degree? It's probably safer than snowboarding and just as challenging.

A FINAL WORD FROM OUR SPONSOR: NURSE KATZ

When I made my Pros and Cons list to see if I wanted to go to nursing school, the Pros outweighed the Cons. Still I was not certain that I was making the right choice, and as I've learned, I had little idea of what being a nurse would really be like. Fortunately, it has worked out very well for me. My final advice to you is that you learn as much as you can about what nursing is, determine whether it fits your needs, and realize that, if you do decide to go to nursing school, there will be many moments of doubt and frustration but just as many of excitement and joy.

Being an RN can be as much fun as a three-ring circus; as interesting as discovering the footprints of the oldest human being; as exciting as rafting down the Colorado River; as difficult as trying to answer the question, "What's the meaning of life?"; and as frightening as having your flashlight die in the depths of the Carlsbad Caverns. All this is true—if you want to be a nurse. And that is the final challenge and the reason you picked up this book—do you want to be a nurse? I hope I've helped you answer that question.

Resources

SUGGESTED READINGS

The following list of books, journal articles, and websites is not comprehensive, but it will give you the insight of others besides myself. As for nursing journals, there are hundreds, so I've listed several general ones that can provide both a broader picture of nursing and a classified section to scan for jobs. The websites are fun to browse, and they will give you ideas of what nurses are doing in the areas of practice, research, and teaching.

Websites

There is an immense amount of information on the Internet from and for nurses, although finding it efficiently can be a problem. The list provided here gives the important sites from which you'll find information on just about everything, including job postings, tips on interviewing and resumés, schools, the NCLEX examination, financial aid, general health, what other nurses are concerned about via chat rooms, and enough legislative information to keep you busy writing letters or e-mailing your senators and representatives.

Information on Nursing Careers

Johnson and Johnson: *Discover Nursing*
www.discovernursing.com
This is one of the best sites to find out more about nursing. The Discover Nursing campaign is sponsored by the Johnson and Johnson Company to promote the career of nursing. Their website is extensive, and you can read about the careers of real nurses including men, nurses with disabilities, and nursing students. The content is divided into four sections: (1) Who, (2) What, (3) Why, and (4) How.

CollegeBoard.com: *Majors and Career Central*
www.collegeboard.com/student/csearch/majors_careers/index.html
CollegeBoard.com is a commercial company specializing in college preparation. The site has links to all kinds of majors, including nursing and advanced practice nursing. You will find a brief description of prerequisites and highlights of the career.

National Student Nurses Association (NSNA)
www.nsna.org
This is the place to go to see the world of nursing from a student's perspective. It contains information on all aspects of nursing, from education to career.

The American Assembly for Men in Nursing
www.aamn.org
This site has links to featured stories about topics that range from men in nursing to information on men's health. You must visit this site to learn more about the importance of men in nursing.

National League for Nursing (NLN): *Resources for Students*
http://www.nln.org/Careers/resources.htm
This section of the NLN website includes links to other good sites, financial aid information sites, and links to sites for international students.

The American Association of Colleges of Nursing (AACN): *Your Nursing Career*
www.aacn.nche.edu/Education/nurse_ed/careerresources.htm
The AACN website is a good place to go to learn more about nursing and related issues. The student section is aimed at nursing students, but going to the subsection

titled, "Your Nursing Career," will lead you to abundant, up-to-date information about nursing. Examples are: "Your Nursing Career: A Look at the Facts" and "Financial Aid Information for Prospective and Current Nursing Students."

Indian Health Service (IHS)
www.ihs.gov
The Indian Health Service website supplies information on both health careers and scholarships. The Indian Health Service (IHS), a federal health program for American Indians and Alaska Natives, provides clinic and hospital care in the United States to enrolled members of a recognized tribe. The IHS is divided into regions (for example, the largest region is the Navajo, the second largest is Oklahoma, and the third largest is the Portland area, which serves Oregon, Washington, and Idaho).

Careers in the Military: *Registered Nurses*
www.careersinthemilitary.com/index.cfm?fuseaction=main.careerdetail&mc_id=120
This site details information on military programs and health services careers in nursing.

American Nurses Association (ANA)
www.nursingworld.org
The ANA website, NursingWorld, includes all kinds of association news, health care updates, publications, and career information. It also includes international nursing opportunities, a legislative branch, state organizations, educational offerings, the *On-line Journal of Issues in Nursing* (one new topic is chosen for each issue), and ethnic and minority fellowship sources.

Bernard Hodes Group: *Nursing Voices: The Stories*
www.hodes.com/industries/healthcare/features/nursingvoices/readstories.asp
From the Bernard Hodes Group website, you will read stories about being a nurse from real RNs, both men and women.

Career Voyages
www.careervoyages.gov/healthcare-main.cfm
The U.S. Department of Labor website has short videos for all high-demand health careers. If you want more information about other health care professions, this might be a site to visit. The site is not nearly as good as the Discover Nursing site. A criticism I have is that they refer to nursing as an occupation, whereas physicians, pharmacists, occupational therapists, and some others are called professions.

Futures in Nursing
www.FuturesInNursing.org/
Although sponsored by the Pennsylvania Higher Education Foundation, this website is not state specific. You will find "Nursing Basics," "Career Planning," "Higher Education," "Student Aid," and links to other nursing sites.

Nursing Spectrum's Student Corner
www.nursingspectrum.com/StudentsCorner/CareersInNursing/
Read about different things you can do in nursing. You can read about being a trauma nurse or a hospital CEO. There is a great section on "Career Alternatives." This includes:
- Entrepreneur/consultant
- Flight nurse

- Forensic nurse
- Holistic nurse
- Medical editor/writer
- Military nursing
- Nursing informatics
- Parish nurse
- Pharm/med sales
- Research nurse
- Travel nurse

Nurse Zone's Student Nurse Center
www.nursezone.com/student_nurse_center/default.asp
This is a commercial site sponsored by various health care organizations. It has a section for students that includes financial aid information, how to select a school, and other student friendly tips.

Nurses for a Healthier Tomorrow: *Career Information*
http://nursesource.org/nursing_careers.html
This section of the website includes information on specialty areas in nursing, applying to nursing school, and the differences between the different nursing degrees (Diploma, ADN, BSN).

Choose Nursing
www.choosenursing.com/
Choose Nursing is sponsored by the Coalition for Nursing Careers in California, but much of the information is not state specific. You can read the online stories of nursing students and nurses.

Global Health Council
www.globalhealth.org/
If you are interested in international health, visit this private nonprofit organization's site. It will give you information on current international health issues, opportunities for student networks (undergraduate and graduate students), and links to overseas job opportunities.

Office of Minority Health, U.S. Department of Health and Human Services
www.omhrc.gov/
This site provides information on minority health issues, funding opportunities, conferences, legislative action in Congress, publications, useful information links, and other information. It also includes the standards for cultural competency.

Diversity Rx
www.diversityrx.org/HTML/DIVRX.htm
This site promotes language and cultural competence to improve the quality of health care for minority, immigrant, and ethnically diverse communities.

Information on Going to College
Campus Blues
www.campusblues.com/
Campus Blues is a commercial site that focuses on mental health issues connected to campus life. Following is a list of the types of things Campus Blues covers.

- Bill Keefe Founder, CampusBlues.com: *What's the Point? I'm Only 18!*
- Dr. Gregory Hall: *Myths and Facts About the College Experience*
- University of Cincinnati Psychological Services Center: *Academic Problems*
- Susan Fee: *Do Best Friends Make Best Roommates?*
- Grayson P, Meilman P: *Fitting In*
- Susan Fee: *Dealing With Stress: 25 Tips*
- Boyum, D, and the University of Wisconsin-Eau Clair Counseling: *Taking the Worry Out of Anxiety*
- *What Type of Eater Are You? Take The Quiz!*

High School Blues
www.highschoolblues.com/
A similar site discusses high school problems. Although the site lists specific high schools, you can go into any of them and find articles about mental health–related issues.

Kaplan Educational Centers
www.kaplan.com
You can find out about business, law, medicine, and nursing specialties, as well as other general career information such as resumé writing, interview skills, financial aid, college entrance exams, and graduate school. Under "Nursing", there is a career path with examples of types of degrees (ADN, BSN, MSN) and job opportunities for each.

Books and Websites: Information on Scholarships and Financial Aid

AmeriCorps
www.americorps.org/
Also referred to as the Corporation for National and Community Service, the AmeriCorps website provides full-time awards in return for community service work. You can work before, during, or after your college education and use the award either to pay current school expenses or to repay loans.

Anna Leider: *Loans and Grants from Uncle Sam: Am I Eligible and for How Much?* ed 13, 2006, Octameron Associates, Alexandria, Virginia
I love this book! It's short and organized and therefore, to my mind, easy to use. The only disadvantage is that it covers only government loans, but that's where you will probably be looking. However, don't forget nongovernmental sources of aid (covered by other sources on this list).

National Health Service Corps
http://nhsc.bhpr.hrsa.gov
This site may be of interest if you plan to pursue graduate education. They will pay for your tuition if you qualify and agree to work in a federally designated under-served area for an agreed-upon length of time.

Peterson's *College Money Handbook* (annual, Peterson's Guides)
Published each year by Peterson's, it can be found in the library reference section. It contains information on 1700 colleges and sources for financial aid.

The Foundation of the National Student Nurses' Association (NSNA), Inc.
www.nsna.org/foundation/index.asp

The NSNA foundation is a good source to check for financial aid and for other information about being a nursing student. Check their website to find all kinds of nursing student advice, the Code of Ethics, conference announcements, career center, and chapter links, additional NCLEX review, and much more.

Federal Student Aid Information Center
http://studentaid.ed.gov/
U.S. Department of Education
1-800-4-FED-AID (800-433-3243)
This website provides a wealth of information and links to the standard guide used by all students seeking government loans, *Funding Education Beyond High School: The Guide to Federal Student Aid*. It explains the different types and what to do to apply for them. The 800 number gives you general information on loans and updates on specific lender information in your area.

• • •

Other sources to investigate for requesting financial aid include community organizations such as the YWCA, 4-H Club, Elks, Kiwanis, Jaycees, Chamber of Commerce, and Girl or Boy Scouts; religious organizations; private foundations; your current place of employment; and labor unions.

Nursing Journals: Print and Online
The American Nurse: The Official Publication of the American Nurses Association (ANA)
www.nursingworld.org/tan/
No other publication gives you a better look quickly at what is happening in nursing. Articles cover issues of concern for nurses, actions nurses are taking to solve health care's problems, and legislative matters the ANA is lobbying for. *The American Nurse* is an excellent way to get the "big picture" of nursing, including a classified jobs section, information on grants, and upcoming educational offerings.

American Journal of Nursing
www.nursingcenter.com
The *AJN* comes by subscription. Its website includes information on continuing education for nurses and a career center with work listed by geographic regions. Their annual Career Guide is also found here, with job listings for nurses by specialty area and location.

Books
The following references cover the topics of finding work in nursing, employment outlooks according to government and nursing organizations that predict such things, and guides to help you decide on a career. Again, this list is far from comprehensive. Use it to get started, remember to go to the library and ask the reference librarian for help.

Books on Nursing Schools and Colleges
National League for Nursing: *A Guide to State-Approved Schools of Nursing RN, 2006*, 57th edition, 2006
This is a directory of state-approved schools of nursing offering educational programs that prepare students for RN licensure. It includes all associate degree, diploma, and

baccalaureate programs that conducted programs in nursing education as of October 15, 2005. Graduates of these three types of basic nursing education programs may have differences in preparation, but all are eligible to take the examination that leads to RN licensure. The book includes many other features related to going to school.

Peterson, T., and Krakowski, J. editors: *Peterson's Guide to Nursing Programs 2006,* 2006, Peterson's Guides
www.petersons.com/nursing/ug_code/ug_start.asp
Peterson's Guide has information about baccalaureate and graduate nursing programs in the United States and Canada. It covers topics such as financial aid, entrance requirements, and different characteristics of programs (for example, if they have distance learning options). The guide also has ideas for how to select a school, information for international students, and links to scholarships.

Books or Reports on Health Care Issues and Policy

Institute of Medicine, Board on Health Care Services: *Health Professions Education: a Bridge to Quality,* 2003, National Academies Press
http://fermat.nap.edu/books/0309087236/html
The Institute of Medicine (IOM) is a gold mine for evidence-based information on health care and health care professions. If you want to explore the bigger picture of health care and get an idea of the trends for the future, start reading. Try *Health Professions Education: A Bridge to Quality.* It will tell you everything about what kinds of health professionals we need and in what areas they need to be educated to improve the quality of health care. The website will take you to the table of contents, where you can click on links to read anything you want. A very nice feature is a "skim" button. Press this and you will get the chapter highlights.

Institute of Medicine, Committee on Institutional and Policy-Level Strategies for Increasing Diversity of the U.S. Healthcare Workforce: *In the Nation's Compelling Interest: Ensuring Diversity in the Health Care Workforce,* 2004, National Academies Press)
http://newton.nap.edu/catalog/10885.html#toc
This is a book I really like. It includes wonderful quotes such as this from the executive summary:

> *Increasing racial and ethnic diversity among health professionals is important because evidence indicates that diversity is associated with improved access to care for racial and ethnic minority patients, greater patient choice and satisfaction, and better educational experiences for health professions students, among many other benefits.*

Books on Nursing

National Nurses in Business Association: *How I Became a Nurse Entrepreneur: Tales from 50 Nurses in Business,* 1998, Power Publications
Want to start your own business? If so, this may be a good book for you. It provides real-life information on business possibilities and how 50 nurses became business owners.

Mary O. Mundinger, editor: *The Pfizer Guide: Nursing Career Opportunities,* Columbia University School of Nursing, 2005, Merritt Communications
You should find this in any health sciences library, if not in the public library. Look for updated versions every 4 or 5 years.

Echo Heron: *Tending Lives: Nurses on the Medical Front*, 1998, Ivy Books, New York
In her books, even though they may be a little dated, Heron, an outspoken advocate of nursing, gives you both an insider's look at real nursing and a good read.

Florence Nightingale: *Notes on Nursing: What It Is and Is Not*, 1969, Dover Publications, Minneola, New York
Nightingale, the founder of modern nursing, gives us the original definition of the professional nurse. First published in 1859 (the same year as Darwin's *On the Origin of Species*), it is fascinating reading.

Susan Reverby: *Ordered to Care: The Dilemma of American Nursing, 1850–1945* 1987, Cambridge University Press, Cambridge, UK
This includes a history of nursing, women's issues, and working women. It is an excellent book to read to gain an understanding of problems faced by nurses today.

O'Lynn, C.E., & Tranbarger, R.E. (Eds.). (2006). *Men in nursing: History, challenges, and opportunities.* New York: Springer Publishing Company.

Tarcher, S.B. (2005). *Nursing America: One year behind the nursing stations of an inner city hospital.*

Karels, C. (2005). *Cooked: An inner city nursing memoir.* (2nd ed.). Hackensack, NJ: Arcania Press.

Winstead-Fry, P. (2005). *Ordinary miracles in nursing.* Sudbury, MA: Jones and Bartlett Publishers.

Nelson, S., & Gordon, S. (Eds.). (2006). *Nursing against the odds: How health care cost cutting, media stereotypes, and medical hubris undermine nurses and patient care (The culture and politics of health care work).* Ithaca, NY: ILR Press.

Satterly, F. (2003) *Where have all the nurses gone? The impact of the nursing shortage on American healthcare.* Amherst, NY: Prometheus Books.

Buresh, B., & Gordon, S. (2006). *From silence to voice: What nurses know and must communicate to the public.* (2nd ed.). Ithaca, NY: ILR Press.

Benner, P. (2001). *From novice to expert: Excellence and power in clinical nursing practice.* (commemorative ed.). Upper Saddle River, NJ: Prentice Hall.

• • •

For other titles, check the website of the American Association for the History of Nursing: (http://aahn.org).

To Do: Observe Nurses in Action

As far as I know, there is no formal setup for watching nurses on the job, but it can be done. If you don't already know a nurse, perhaps the following sources can hook you up with the right person—but beware of one snag: the new privacy laws (HIPPA regulations):

- *Local Hospital, Home Health Agency, Public Health Department:* Call one of these in your area and ask to speak to either the educational services department, or, if there isn't one, try the director of nursing. Explain that you are interested in nursing as a career and would like to observe an RN at work. They should be able to help you connect with one.
- *Local Nursing School:* Call the admissions office or career placement office and tell them what you want to do (see above). Most universities or colleges with a nursing school will have a nursing adviser who will be thrilled at your request and gladly help you out.

Nursing Organizations

MINORITY NURSING ASSOCIATIONS*

Aboriginal Nurses Association of Canada
12 Stirling Avenue, 3rd Floor
Ottawa, ON K1Y 1P8
www.anac.on.ca/

Asian American/Pacific Islander Nurses Association
400 N. Ingalls, Suite 3160
Ann Arbor, MI 48109-0482
Phone (734) 998-1030
Contact: SeonAe Yeo, President, Seonaeyo@umich.edu
www.aapina.org

The American Assembly for Men in Nursing
11 Cornell Road
Latham, NY 12110-1499
http://aamn.org

Filipino Nurses Online
Filipino Nurses Online is a nonprofit Internet-based organization designed to create a link to all regional divisions of the Philippine Nurses Association located in different parts of the world.
http://www.geocities.com/fil_nsg/

National Alaska Native American Indian Nurses Association
3702 S. Fife St.
Tacoma, WA 98409-7318
Phone/Fax: (888) 566-8773
www.nanainanurses.org/

National Association of Hispanic Nurses
1501 16th St., NW
Washington, DC 20036
Phone: (202) 387-2477
Fax: (202) 483-7183
info@nahnhq.org
www.thehispanicnurses.org

The National Black Nurses Association, Inc.
8630 Fenton St., Suite 330
Silver Spring, MD 20910
Phone: (301) 589-3200
Fax: (301) 589-3223
nbna@erols.com
www.nbna.org/

*Listing adapted from MinorityNurse.com (www.minoritynurse.com/associations/).

National Coalition of Ethnic Minority Nurse Associations
5630 Arch Crest Drive
Los Angeles, CA 90043
Phone: (323) 294-4676
Fax (323) 292-5001
Betwilliam@aol.com
www.ncemna.org

Philippine Nurses Association of America, Inc.
20127 Avenida Pamplona
Cerritos, CA 90703
milavelasquez@att.net
www.pnaa03.org

MINORITY HEALTH ASSOCIATIONS*

Alliance of Minority Medical Associations
The AMMA collectively supports the moral imperative that all individuals are
equally entitled to receive high-quality health care therapies that can improve and
prolong life.
655 15th St., NW
Suite 475A
Washington, DC 20005
Phone: (202) 347-3820 Ext: 5943
info@AllAmericanHealth.org
www.ammaonline.org

American Public Health Association
The American Public Health Association is the oldest and largest organization of
public health professionals in the world, representing more than 50,000 members
from over 50 occupations of public health, including nursing.
800 I St., NW
Washington, DC 20001-3710
Phone: (202) 777-APHA
Fax: (202) 777-2534
www.apha.org

American Samoa Health Services
Regulatory Board
LBJ Tropical Medical Center
Pago Pago, AS 96799
Phone: (684)633-1222
Fax: (684)633-1869
Contact Person: Toaga Atuatasi Seumalo, MS, RN, Executive Secretary
website: N/A

*Listing adapted from MinorityNurse.com (www.minoritynurse.com/associations/).

Asian & Pacific Islander American Health Forum
942 Market St., Suite 200
San Francisco, CA 94102
Phone: (415)954-9988
Fax: (415)954-9999
hforum@apiahf.org
www.apiahf.org

Association of American Indian Physicians
1235 Sovereign Row, Suite C-9
Oklahoma City, OK 73108
Phone: (405) 946-7072
Fax: (405) 946-7651
aaip@ionet.net
www.aaip.com

Association of Asian Pacific Community Health Organizations
1440 Broadway, Suite 510
Oakland, CA 94612
Phone: (510) 272-9536
Fax: (510) 272-0817
www.aapcho.org

Association of American Medical Colleges
2450 N St., NW
Washington, D.C. 20037-1127
Phone: (202) 828-0400
Fax: (202) 828-1120
www.aamc.org/diversity

National Asian Women's Health Organization
250 Montgomery St., Suite 1500
San Francisco, CA 94104
Phone: (415) 989-9747
Fax: (415) 989-9758
nawho@nawho.org
www.nawho.org

National Alliance for Hispanic Health
1501 16th St., NW
Washington, DC 20036-1401
Phone: (202) 387-5000
alliance@hispanichealth.org
www.hispanichealth.org

National Hispanic Medical Association
1411 K St., NW, Suite 1100
Washington, DC 20005
Phone: (202) 628-5895
Fax: (202) 628-5898
www.nhmamd.org

National Indian Health Board
Parklawn Building
Indian Health Service
5600 Fishers Lane
Rockville, MD 20857
www.nihb.org

National Medical Association
(A national association of African-American physicians)
1012 10th St., NW
Washington, D.C. 20001
Phone: (202) 347-1895
Fax: (202) 842-3293
www.nmanet.org

National Minority AIDS Council
1931 13th St., NW
Washington, DC 20009
info@nmac.org
www.nmac.org

Transcultural Nursing Society
The TCNS defines transcultural nursing as "an essential area of study and practice focused on the cultural care beliefs, values and lifeways of people to help them maintain and/or regain their health, or to face death in meaningful ways." The society confers the Certified Transcultural Nurse (CTN) certification.
36600 Schoolcraft Road
Livonia, MI 48150-1173
Phone: (734) 432-5470; toll-free (888) 432-5470
Fax: (734) 432-5463
www.tcns.org

GENERAL ORGANIZATIONS

The following pages are not meant to contain a complete list of all nursing organizations. For others, visit the Internet nursing websites (see Appendix A).

American Nurses Association
600 Maryland Ave. SW, Suite 100 W
Washington, DC 20024-2571
Phone: 1-800-274-4262
www.nursingworld.org

United American Nurses AFL/CIO
The bargaining arm of the ANA for nurses also works on legislative issues such as the following:
• RN Staffing Ratio Bill
• Mandatory Overtime Ban
• Employee Free Choice Act
• Protecting RN Overtime Pay
• TB Respirator Fit Testing

8515 Georgia Ave., Suite 400
Silver Spring, MD 20910
Phone: (301) 628-5118
Fax: (301) 628-5347
UANInfo@UANNurse.org
www.uannurse.org/

Canadian Nurses' Association
50 Driveway
Ottawa, ON
K2P 1E2 Canada
Phone: (613) 237-2133
www.cna-nurses.ca

National League for Nursing
Communications Department
350 Hudson St., 4th Floor
New York, NY 10014
Phone: (212) 989-9393
Center for Career Advancement
Phone: 1-800-669-9656 ext. 143
www.nln.org

National Student Nurses' Association
555 West 57th St., Suite 1325
New York, NY 10019
Phone: (212) 581-2211
www.nsna.org

STATE AND FEDERAL NURSING ASSOCIATIONS

Alabama State Nurses Association (ASNA)
www.alabamanurses.org

Alaska Nurses Association (AaNA)
www.aknurse.org

Arizona Nurses Association (AzNA)
www.aznurse.org

Arkansas Nurses Association (ArNA)
www.arna.org

American Nurses Association California (ANAC)
www.anacalifornia.org

Colorado Nurses Association (CNA)
www.nurses-co.org

Connecticut Nurses' Association (CNA)
www.ctnurses.org

Delaware Nurses Association (DNA)
www.denurses.org

District of Columbia Nurses Association (DCNA)
www.dcna.org

Federal Nurses Association (FedNA)
www.nursingworld.org/FedNA

Florida Nurses Association (FNA)
www.floridanurse.org

Georgia Nurses Association (GNA)
www.georgianurses.org

Hawaii Nurses Association (HNA)
www.hawaiinurses.org

Idaho Nurses Association (INA)
www.nursingworld.org/snas/id

Illinois Nurses Association (INA)
www.illinoisnurses.com

Indiana State Nurses Association (ISNA)
www.indiananurses.org

Iowa Nurses' Association (INA)
www.iowanurses.org

Kansas State Nurses Association (KSNA)
www.nursingworld.org/snas/ks

Kentucky Nurses Association (KNA)
www.kentucky-nurses.org

Louisiana State Nurses Association (LSNA)
www.lsna.org

American Nurses Association Maine (ANA-Maine)
www.anamaine.org

Maryland Nurses Association (MNA)
www.marylandrn.org

Massachusetts Association of Registered Nurses (MARN)
www.marnonline.org

Michigan Nurses Association (MNA)
www.minurses.org

Minnesota Nurses Association (MNA)
www.mnnurses.org

Mississippi Nurses Association (MNA)
www.msnurses.org

The Missouri Nurses Association (MONA)
www.missourinurses.org

Montana Nurses Association (MNA)
www.mtnurses.org

Nebraska Nurses Association (NNA)
http://nursingworld.org/cmas/ne/

Nevada Nurses Association (NNA)
www.nvnurses.org

New Hampshire Nurses' Association (NHNA)
www.NHnurses.org

New Jersey State Nurses Association (NJSNA)
www.njsna.org

New Mexico Nurses Association (NMNA)
www.nmna.org

New York State Nurses Association (NYSNA)
www.nysna.org

North Carolina Nurses Association (NCNA)
www.ncnurses.org

North Dakota Nurses Association (NDNA)
www.ndna.org

Ohio Nurses Association (ONA)
www.ohnurses.org

Oklahoma Nurses Association (ONA)
www.oknurses.com

Oregon Nurses Association (ONA)
www.oregonrn.org

Pennsylvania State Nurses Association (PSNA)
www.panurses.org

Rhode Island State Nurses Association (RISNA)
www.risnarn.org

South Carolina Nurses Association (SCNA)
www.scnurses.org

South Dakota Nurses Association (SDNA)
www.sdnursesassociation.org

Tennessee Nurses Association (TNA)
www.tnaonline.org

Texas Nurses Association (TNA)
www.texasnurses.org

Utah Nurses Association (UNA)
www.utahnurses.org

Vermont State Nurses Association, Inc. (VSNA)
www.vsna-inc.org/

Virginia Nurses Association (VNA)
www.virginianurses.com

Washington State Nurses Association (WSNA)
www.wsna.org

West Virginia Nurses Association (WVNA)
www.wvnurses.org

Wisconsin Nurses Association (WNA)
www.wisconsinnurses.org

Wyoming Nurses Association (WNA)
www.wyonurse.org

STATE BOARDS OF NURSING

Alabama Board of Nursing
770 Washington Avenue
RSA Plaza, Suite 250
Montgomery, AL 36130-3900
Phone: (334) 242-4060
Fax: (334) 242-4360
Contact Person: N. Genell Lee, MSN, JD, RN, Executive Officer
www.abn.state.al.us

Alaska Board of Nursing
550 West Seventh Ave., Suite 1500
Anchorage, AK 99501-3567
Phone: (907) 269-8161
Fax: (907) 269-8196
Contact Person: Dorothy Fulton, MA, RN, Executive Administrator
www.dced.state.ak.us/occ/pnur.htm

Arizona State Board of Nursing
4747 North 7th St., Suite 200
Phoenix, AZ 85014-3653
Phone: (602) 889-5150
Fax: (602) 889-5155
Contact Person: Joey Ridenour, MN, RN, Executive Director
www.azbn.gov

Arkansas State Board of Nursing
University Tower Building
1123 S. University, Suite 800
Little Rock, AR 72204-1619
Phone: (501) 686-2700
Fax: (501) 686-2714
Contact Person: Faith Fields, MSN, RN, Executive Director
www.state.ar.us/nurse

California Board of Registered Nursing
1625 North Market Blvd., Suite N-217
Sacramento, CA 95834-1924
Phone: (916) 322-3350
Fax: (916) 574 -8637
Contact Person: Ruth Ann Terry, MPH, RN, Executive Officer
www.rn.ca.gov

Colorado Board of Nursing
1560 Broadway, Suite 880
Denver, CO 80202
Phone: (303) 894-2430
Fax: (303) 894-2821
Contact Person: Linda Volz, Program Director
www.dora.state.co.us/nursing

Connecticut Board of Examiners for Nursing
Dept. of Public Health
410 Capitol Avenue, MS# 13PHO
P.O. Box 340308
Hartford, CT 06134-0328
Phone: (860) 509-7624
Fax: (860) 509-7553
Contact Person: Jan Wojick, Board Liaison
Nancy L. Bafundo, BSN, MS, RN, Board President
www.state.ct.us/dph/

Delaware Board of Nursing
861 Silver Lake Blvd.
Cannon Building, Suite 203
Dover, DE 19904
Phone: (302) 739.4522
Fax: (302) 739.2711
Contact Person: Iva Boardman, MSN, RN, Executive Director
www.professionallicensing.state.de.us/boards/nursing/index.shtml

District of Columbia Board of Nursing
Department of Health
717 14th St., NW, Suite 600
Washington, DC 20005
Phone: (202) 724-4900
Fax: (202) 727-8241
Contact Person: Karen Scipio-Skinner MSN, RN, Executive Director
www.dchealth.dc.gov/

Florida Board of Nursing
Florida Board of Nursing
4052 Bald Cypress Way
BIN C02
Tallahassee, FL 32399
Phone: (850) 245-4125
Fax: (850) 245-4172
Contact Person: Vacant, Executive Director
http://www.doh.state.fl.us/mqa/nursing/

Georgia State Board of Licensed Practical Nurses
237 Coliseum Drive
Macon, GA 31217-3858
Phone: (478) 2071640
Fax: (478) 207-1633
Contact Person: Brig Zimmerman, Executive Director
http://www.sos.state.ga.us/plb/lpn

Georgia Board of Nursing
237 Coliseum Drive
Macon, GA 31217-3858
Phone: (478) 207-1640
Fax: (478) 207-1660
Contact Person: Sylvia Bond, RN MSN, MBA, Executive Director
http://www.sos.state.ga.us/plb/rn

Guam Board of Nurse Examiners
Regular mailing address
P.O. Box 2816
Hagatna, Guam 96932
Phone: (671) 735-7406
(671) 725-7411
Fax: (671) 735-7413
Contact Person: Lillian Perez-Posadas, Interim Executive Officer

Hawaii Board of Nursing
King Kalakaua Building
335 Merchant St., 3rd Floor
Honolulu, HI 96813
Phone: (808) 586-3000
Fax: (808) 586-2689
Contact Person: Kathleen Yokouchi, MBA, BBA, BA, Executive Officer
www.hawaii.gov/dcca/areas/pvl/boards/nursing

Idaho Board of Nursing
280 N. 8th St., Suite 210
P.O. Box 83720
Boise, ID 83720
Phone: (208) 334-3110
Fax: (208) 334-3262
Contact Person: Sandra Evans, MA, Ed, RN, Executive Director
www2.state.id.us/ibn/

Illinois Department of Professional Regulation
James R. Thompson Center
100 West Randolph, Suite 9-300
Chicago, IL 60601
Phone: (312) 814-2715
Fax: (312) 814-3145
Contact Person: Vacant, Nursing Act Coordinator
www.dpr.state.il.us/

Indiana State Board of Nursing
Professional Licensing Agency
402 W. Washington St., Room W072
Indianapolis, IN 46204
Phone: (317) 234-2043
Fax: (317) 233-4236
Contact Person: Tonja Thompson, Director of Nursing
www.in.gov/pla/

Iowa Board of Nursing
RiverPoint Business Park
400 S.W. 8th St., Suite B
Des Moines, IA 50309-4685
Phone: (515) 281-3255
Fax: (515) 281-4825
Contact Person: Lorinda Inman, MSN, RN, Executive Director
www.state.ia.us/government/nursing/

Kansas State Board of Nursing
Landon State Office Building
900 S.W. Jackson, Suite 1051
Topeka, KS 66612
Phone: (785) 296-4929
Fax: (785) 296-3929
Contact Person: Mary Blubaugh, MSN, RN, Executive Administrator
www.ksbn.org/

Kentucky Board of Nursing
312 Whittington Parkway, Suite 300
Louisville, KY 40222
Phone: (502) 429-3300
Fax: (502) 429-3311
Contact Person: Charlotte F. Beason, Ed.D, RN, CNAA, Executive Director
www.kbn.ky.gov/

Louisiana State Board of Nursing
3510 N. Causeway Blvd., Suite 601
Metairie, LA 70002
Phone: (225) 763-3570 or (225) 763-3577
Fax: (225) 763-3580
Temporary Address:
5207 Essen Lane, Suite 6
Baton Rouge, LA 70809
Phone: (504) 838-5332
Fax: (504) 838-5349
Contact Person: Barbara Morvant, MN, RN, Executive Director
www.lsbn.state.la.us

Maine State Board of Nursing
Regular mailing address
158 State House Station
Augusta, ME 04333
Phone: (207) 287-1133
Fax: (207) 287-1149
Contact Person: Myra Broadway, JD, MS, RN, Executive Director
www.maine.gov/boardofnursing/

Maryland Board of Nursing
4140 Patterson Avenue
Baltimore, MD 21215
Phone: (410) 585-1900
Fax: (410) 358-3530
Contact Person: Donna Dorsey, MS, RN, Executive Director
www.mbon.org/main.php

Massachusetts Board of Registration in Nursing
Commonwealth of Massachusetts
239 Causeway St., Second Floor
Boston, MA 02114
Phone: (617) 973-0800
(800) 414-0168
Fax: (617) 973-0984
Contact Person: Rula Faris Harb, MS, RN, Executive Director
www.mass.gov/dpl/boards/rn/

Michigan/DCH/Bureau of Health Professions
Ottawa Towers North
611 W. Ottawa, 1st Floor
Lansing, MI 48933
Phone: (517) 335-0918
Fax: (517) 373-2179
Contact Person: Diane Lewis, MBA, BA, Policy Manager for Licensing Division
www.michigan.gov/healthlicense

Minnesota Board of Nursing
2829 University Ave. SE
Minneapolis, MN 55414
Phone: (612) 617-2270
Fax: (612) 617-2190
Contact Person: Shirley Brekken, MS, RN, Executive Director
www.nursingboard.state.mn.us/

Mississippi Board of Nursing
1935 Lakeland Drive, Suite B
Jackson, MS 39216-5014
Phone: (601) 987-4188
Fax: (601) 364-2352
Contact Person: Delia Owens, RN, JD, Executive Director
www.msbn.state.ms.us/

Missouri State Board of Nursing
3605 Missouri Blvd.
P.O. Box 656
Jefferson City, MO 65102-0656
Phone: (573) 751-0681
Fax: (573) 751-0075
Contact Person: Lori Scheidt, BS, Executive Director
http://pr.mo.gov/nursing.asp

Montana State Board of Nursing
301 South Park
P.O. Box 200513
Helena, MT 59620-0513
Phone: (406) 841-2340
Fax: (406) 841-2305
Contact Person: Sandra Dickenson, Executive Director
www.discoveringmontana.com/dli/bsd/license/bsd_boards/nur_board/board_page.asp

Nebraska Department of Health and Human Services Regulation and Licensure
Nursing and Nursing Support
301 Centennial Mall South
Lincoln, NE 68509-4986
Phone: (402) 471-4376
Fax: (402) 471-1066
Contact Person: Charlene Kelly, PhD, RN, Executive Director
    Nursing and Nursing Support
www.hhs.state.ne.us/crl/nursing/nursingindex.htm

Nevada State Board of Nursing
5011 Meadowood Mall #201
Reno, NV 89502-6547
Phone: (775) 688-2620
Fax: (775) 688-2628
Contact Person: Debra Scott, MS, RN, Executive Director
www.nursingboard.state.nv.us/

New Hampshire Board of Nursing
21 South Fruit St., Suite 16
Concord, NH 03301-2341
Phone: (603) 271-2323
Fax: (603) 271-6605
Contact Person: Margaret Walker, MBA, BSN, RN, Executive Director
www.state.nh.us/nursing/

New Jersey Board of Nursing
P.O. Box 45010
124 Halsey St., 6th Floor
Newark, NJ 07101
Phone: (973) 504-6430
Fax: (973) 648-3481
Contact Person: George Hebert, Executive Director
www.state.nj.us/lps/ca/medical/nursing.htm

New Mexico Board of Nursing
6301 Indian School Road, NE
Suite 710
Albuquerque, NM 87110
Phone: (505) 841-8340
Fax: (505) 841-8347
Contact Person: Allison Kozeliski, RN, Executive Director
www.bon.state.nm.us/index.html

New York State Board of Nursing
Education Bldg.
89 Washington Ave.
2nd Floor West Wing
Albany, NY 12234
Phone: (518) 474-3817, Ext. 280
Fax: (518) 474-3706
Contact Person: Barbara Zittel, PhD, RN, Executive Secretary
www.nysed.gov/prof/nurse.htm

North Carolina Board of Nursing
3724 National Drive, Suite 201
Raleigh, NC 27602
Phone: (919) 782-3211
Fax: (919) 781-9461
Contact Person: Polly Johnson, MSN, RN, Executive Director
www.ncbon.com/

North Dakota Board of Nursing
919 South 7th St., Suite 504
Bismarck, ND 58504
Phone: (701) 328-9777
Fax: (701) 328-9785
Contact Person: Constance Kalanek, PhD, RN, Executive Director
www.ndbon.org/

Northern Mariana Islands
Commonwealth Board of Nurse Examiners
P.O. Box 501458
Saipan, MP 96950
Phone: (670) 664-4812
Fax: (670) 664-4813
Contact Person: Rosa M. Tuleda, Associate Director of Public Health & Nursing

Ohio Board of Nursing
17 South High St., Suite 400
Columbus, OH 43215-3413
Phone: (614) 466-3947
Fax: (614) 466-0388
Contact Person: Betsy J. Houchen, RN, MS, JD, Executive Director
www.nursing.ohio.gov/

Oklahoma Board of Nursing
2915 N. Classen Blvd., Suite 524
Oklahoma City, OK 73106
Phone: (405) 962-1800
Fax: (405) 962-1821
Contact Person: Kimberly Glazier, M.Ed., RN, Executive Director
www.youroklahoma.com/nursing

Oregon State Board of Nursing
800 NE Oregon St., Box 25
Suite 465
Portland, OR 97232
Phone: (971) 673-0685
Fax: (971) 673-0684
Contact Person: Joan Bouchard, MN, RN, Executive Director
www.osbn.state.or.us/

Pennsylvania State Board of Nursing
P.O. Box 2649
Harrisburg, PA 17105-2649
Phone: (717) 783-7142
Fax: (717) 783-0822
Contact Person: Laurette D. Keiser, RN, MSN, Executive Secretary/Section Chief
www.dos.state.pa.us/bpoa/cwp/view.asp?a=1104&q=432869

Puerto Rico
Commonwealth of Puerto Rico
Board of Nurse Examiners
Mailing Address:
Office of Regulations and Certifications of Health Professionals
P.O. Box 10200
Santurce, PR 00908-0200
Phone: (787) 725-7506
Fax: (787) 725-7903
Contact Person: Roberto Figueroa, RN, MSN, Executive Director of the Office of
  Regulations and Certifications of Health Care Professions

**Rhode Island Board of Nurse
Registration and Nursing Education**
105 Cannon Building
Three Capitol Hill
Providence, RI 02908
Phone: (401) 222-5700
Fax: (401) 222-3352
Contact Person: Vacant, Executive Officer
www.health.ri.gov/

South Carolina State Board of Nursing
Mailing Address
P.O. Box 12367
Columbia, SC 29211
Phone: (803) 896-4550
Fax: (803) 896-4525
Contact Person: Joan K. Bainer, RN, MN, CNA BC, Administrator
www.llr.state.sc.us/pol/nursing

South Dakota Board of Nursing
4305 South Louise Ave., Suite 201
Sioux Falls, SD 57106-3115
Phone: (605) 362-2760
Fax: (605) 362-2768
Contact Person: Gloria Damgaard, RN, MS, Executive Secretary
www.state.sd.us/doh/nursing/

Tennessee State Board of Nursing
425 Fifth Ave. North
1st Floor - Cordell Hull Building
Nashville, TN 37247
Phone: (615) 532-5166
Fax: (615) 741-7899
Contact Person: Elizabeth Lund, MSN, RN, Executive Director
www.tennessee.gov/health

Texas Board of Nurse Examiners
333 Guadalupe, Suite 3-460
Austin, TX 78701
Phone: (512) 305-7400
Fax: (512) 305-7401
Contact Person: Katherine Thomas, MN, RN, Executive Director
www.bne.state.tx.us/

Utah State Board of Nursing
Heber M. Wells Bldg., 4th Floor
160 East 300 South
Salt Lake City, UT 84111
Phone: (801) 530-6628
Fax: (801) 530-6511
Contact Person: Laura Poe, MS, RN, Executive Administrator
www.dopl.utah.gov/licensing/nurse.html

Vermont State Board of Nursing
81 River St.
Heritage Building
Montpelier, VT 05609-1106
Phone: (802) 828-2396
Fax: (802) 828-2484
Contact Person: Anita Ristau, MS, RN, Executive Director
www.vtprofessionals.org/opr1/nurses/

Virgin Islands Board of Nurse Licensure
P.O. Box 4247, Veterans Drive Station
St. Thomas, VI 00803
Phone: (340) 776-7397
Fax: (340) 777-4003
Contact Person: Vacant, Executive Secretary

Virginia Board of Nursing
6603 West Broad St.
5th Floor
Richmond, VA 23230-1712
Phone: (804) 662-9909
Fax: (804) 662-9512
Contact Person: Jay Douglas, RN, MSM, CSAC, Executive Director
www.dhp.virginia.gov/nursing/

Washington State Nursing Care Quality
Assurance Commission
Department of Health
HPQA #6
310 Israel Rd. SE
Tumwater, WA 98501-7864
Phone: (360) 236-4700
Fax: (360) 236-4738
Contact Person: Paula Meyer, MSN, RN, Executive Director
https://fortress.wa.gov/doh/hpqa1/hps6/Nursing/default.htm

West Virginia Board of Examiners for Registered Professional Nurses
101 Dee Drive
Charleston, WV 25311
Phone: (304) 558-3596
Fax: (304) 558-3666
Contact Person: Laura Rhodes, MSN, RN, Executive Director
www.wvrnboard.com/

Wisconsin Department of Regulation and Licensing
1400 E. Washington Ave., RM 173
Madison, WI 53708
Phone: (608) 266-0145
Fax: (608) 261-7083
Contact Person: Kimberly Nania, PhD, MA, BS, Director,
    Bureau of Health Service Professions
www.drl.state.wi.us/

Wyoming State Board of Nursing
1810 Pioneer Ave.
Cheyenne, WY 82001
Phone: (307) 777-7601
Fax: (307) 777-3519
Contact Person: Cheryl Lynn Koski, MN, RN, CS, Executive Director
http://nursing.state.wy.us/

SPECIALTY ORGANIZATIONS

To access the specialty nursing organizations listed below, visit the following URL on the website for Sigma Theta Tau, Honor Society of Nursing, and click on the organization name: **www.nursingsociety.org/career/nursing_orgs.html.**
Aboriginal Nurses Association of Canada
Academy of Medical Surgical Nurses
Air and Surface Transport Nurses Association
American Academy of Ambulatory Care Nursing
American Academy of Nurse Practitioners
American Academy of Nursing
American Assembly for Men in Nursing
American Association for the History of Nursing
American Association of Colleges of Nursing
American Association of Critical Care Nurses
American Association of Diabetes Educators
American Association of Legal Nurse Consultants
American Association of Managed Care Nurses
American Association of Neuroscience Nurses
American Association of Nurse Anesthetists
American Association of Nurse Attorneys
American Association of Occupational Health Nurses
American Association of Office Nurses
American Association of Spinal Cord Injury Nurses
American College of Nurse-Midwives
American College of Nurse Practitioners
American Holistic Nurses' Association
American Nephrology Nurses' Association
American Nurses Association
American Nurses Foundation
American Nursing Informatics Association
American Organization of Nurse Executives
American Psychiatric Nurses Association
American Public Health Association—Public Health Nursing
American Radiological Nurses Association
American Society of Ophthalmic Registered Nurses
American Society of PeriAnesthesia Nurses
American Society of Plastic Surgical Nurses
Association of Camp Nurses
Association of Nurses in AIDS Care
Association of periOperative Registered Nurses (AORN)
Association of Pediatric Oncology Nurses
Association of Rehabilitation Nurses

Association of Women's Health, Obstetric and Neonatal Nurses
CARING: Capitol Area Roundtable on Informatics in Nursing
Commission on Graduates of Foreign Nursing Schools
Dermatology Nurses Association
Development Disabilities Nurses Association
Emergency Nurses Association
Health Ministries Association
Home Healthcare Nurses Association
Hospice and Palliative Nurses Association
International Council of Nurses
International Association of Forensic Nurses
International Nurses Society on Addictions
International Transplant Nurses Society
International Society for Psychiatric-Mental Health Nurses
Intravenous Nurses Society
National Alaska Native American Indian Nurses Association
National Association of Clinical Nurse Specialists
National Association of Geriatric Nursing Assistants
National Association of Hispanic Nurses
National Association of Neonatal Nurses
National Association of Nurse Massage Therapists
National Association of Orthopaedic Nurses
National Association of Pediatric Nurse Practitioners
National Association of School Nurses
National Black Nurses Association
National Council of State Boards of Nursing
National Gerontological Nursing Association
National League for Nursing
National Nursing Staff Development Organization
National Organization of Nurse Practitioner Faculties
National Rural Health Association
Nurse Practitioner Associates for Continuing Education
Nursing Information Systems Council of New England
Nursing Standard
National Student Nurses Association
Oncology Nursing Society
Pediatric Endocrinology Nursing Association
Philippine Nurses Association of America
Preventive Cardiovascular Nurses Association
Society of Gastroenterology Nurses and Associates
Society of Otorhinolaryngology and Head-Neck Nurses
Society of Pediatric Nurses
Society of Trauma Nurses
Society of Urologic Nurses and Associates
Society for Vascular Nursing
State Nurses Associations
Transcultural Nursing Society
Wound, Ostomy and Continence Nurses Society